SUPER EASY ANTI-INFLAMMATORY DIET

Delicious and Simple Stress-free Recipe to Reduce Inflammation and Heal Your Body

Melvin V. Serrano

Table Of Contents

08 Sweet Treats Recipes

Introduction

Charlotte had always been a go-getter, juggling a demanding job, an active social life, and a love for travel. But recently, she had started to feel different—constantly fatigued, dealing with unexplained aches, and struggling with digestive issues. A visit to her doctor revealed that she was dealing with chronic inflammation, a condition that had been silently affecting her health. Determined to regain her vitality, Charlotte dived into research and discovered the anti-inflammatory diet. However, she was initially overwhelmed by the plethora of information and complex recipes she encountered. She needed something practical and straightforward, something that fit into her busy lifestyle without adding stress.

That's when she stumbled upon "Super Easy Anti-Inflammatory Diet." The title promised simplicity and ease, exactly what she needed. With a mix of curiosity and hope, Charlotte decided to give it a try.

The first week was a revelation. The recipes were not only simple but also delicious.

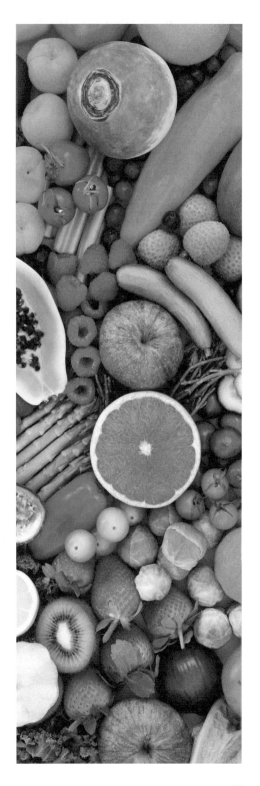

She found herself looking forward to meals rather than dreading the kitchen. Mornings started with refreshing smoothies and nourishing breakfasts, while lunches and dinners were wholesome yet quick to prepare. Within days, Charlotte noticed a change. Her energy levels began to rise, the persistent aches faded, and her digestion improved significantly.

As the weeks went by, Charlotte realized that this wasn't just a diet; it was a lifestyle change. She felt more in tune with her body, more connected to the food she ate. The inflammation reduced, and she felt lighter, both physically and mentally. Her skin glowed, her mind was clearer, and she had a renewed zest for life.

"Super Easy Anti-Inflammatory Diet" became more than just a cookbook for Charlotte; it was a companion on her journey to wellness. It showed her that healthy eating didn't have to be complicated or time-consuming. It could be easy, enjoyable, and incredibly rewarding.

Charlotte's story is a testament to the transformative power of simple, wholesome food. This book is for anyone seeking a similar journey.

Chapter 1: Understanding Inflammation

Inflammation is a natural and vital part of the body's immune response. When your body senses injury, infection, or harmful stimuli, it triggers inflammation to protect itself and initiate the healing process. This response is characterized by redness, warmth, swelling, and pain. In the short term, inflammation is beneficial; it helps wounds heal and fights off infections.

However, not all inflammation is good. Chronic inflammation, which persists for months or even years, can have detrimental effects on your health. Unlike acute inflammation that resolves after the healing process, chronic inflammation continues to attack your body's tissues even when there is no apparent injury or infection. This prolonged state of inflammation can contribute to a variety of health issues, including:

Heart Disease: Chronic inflammation can damage the inner lining of the arteries, leading to the buildup of plaque and increasing the risk of heart attacks and strokes.

Diabetes: Inflammation can interfere with insulin's ability to regulate blood sugar levels, leading to insulin resistance and, eventually, type 2 diabetes.

Arthritis: Conditions like rheumatoid arthritis are driven by chronic inflammation in the joints, causing pain, stiffness, and swelling.

Digestive Disorders: Inflammatory bowel diseases like Crohn's disease and ulcerative colitis are marked by ongoing inflammation in the digestive tract.

Cancer: Chronic inflammation can contribute to the development and progression of certain cancers by damaging DNA and promoting abnormal cell growth.

Mental Health: Emerging research suggests that chronic inflammation may be linked to mental health conditions such as depression and anxiety.

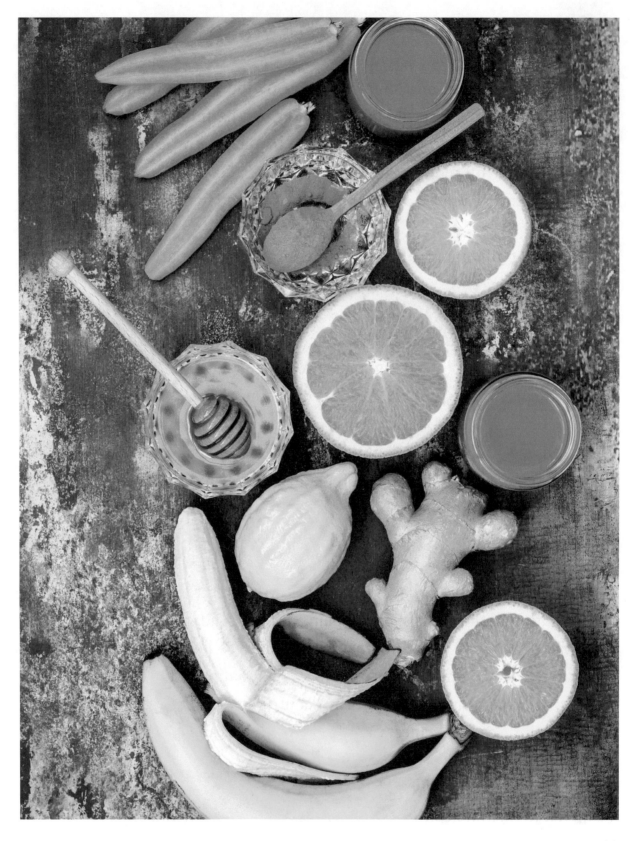

Causes of Chronic Inflammation

Chronic inflammation can be caused by a number of factors, including:
Poor Diet: Diets high in processed foods, refined sugars, and unhealthy fats can promote inflammation.
Lack of Exercise: Regular physical activity helps regulate the immune system and reduce inflammation.
Stress: Chronic stress can trigger inflammatory responses in the body.
Environmental Toxins: Exposure to pollutants and chemicals can contribute to inflammation.
Infections: Persistent infections can keep the immune system in a state of constant alert.

The Role of Diet in Managing Inflammation

One of the most powerful tools to combat chronic inflammation lies at the end of your fork. An anti-inflammatory diet focuses on whole, nutrient-dense foods that can help reduce inflammation and support overall health. Important elements of a diet that reduces inflammation include:

Fruits and Vegetables: Rich in antioxidants and phytonutrients, they help neutralize harmful free radicals and reduce inflammation.
Healthy Fats: Omega-3 fatty acids found in fatty fish, flaxseeds, and walnuts have strong anti-inflammatory properties.
Whole Grains: Unlike refined grains, whole grains retain their nutrients and fiber, which help regulate the body's inflammatory response.
Lean Proteins: Sources like poultry, beans, and legumes provide essential amino acids without the inflammatory effects of processed meats.
Herbs and Spices: Turmeric, ginger, garlic, and other spices contain compounds that can help fight inflammation

Benefits of an Anti-Inflammatory Diet

An anti-inflammatory diet is more than just a way of eating; it's a powerful approach to improving your overall health and well-being. By focusing on nutrient-dense, whole foods that help combat inflammation, you can experience a wide range of health benefits. Here are some key advantages of adopting an anti-inflammatory diet:

1. Reduced Risk of Chronic Diseases

Chronic inflammation is a major contributor to various diseases, including heart disease, diabetes, cancer, and Alzheimer's disease. By minimizing inflammation, an anti-inflammatory diet can help lower the risk of developing these conditions. For example, omega-3 fatty acids found in fatty fish have been shown to reduce the risk of heart disease by lowering triglycerides and blood pressure.

2. Improved Digestive Health

Inflammation in the gut can lead to digestive disorders such as irritable bowel syndrome (IBS), Crohn's disease, and ulcerative colitis. An anti-inflammatory diet, rich in fiber from fruits, vegetables, and whole grains, supports a healthy gut microbiome, promotes regular bowel movements, and reduces symptoms of digestive discomfort.

3. Enhanced Mental Clarity and Mood

Emerging research suggests a strong connection between chronic inflammation and mental health conditions such as depression and anxiety. Foods that fight inflammation, like leafy greens, berries, and nuts, can support brain health and improve mood. The antioxidants and healthy fats in these foods protect brain cells from oxidative stress and inflammation, leading to better cognitive function and emotional well-being.

4. Joint Pain Relief

For those suffering from arthritis or other inflammatory joint conditions, an anti-inflammatory diet can provide significant relief. Foods like turmeric, ginger, and fatty fish contain anti-inflammatory compounds that can reduce joint pain and stiffness, improving mobility and quality of life.

5. Better Skin Health

Chronic inflammation can manifest in the skin, leading to conditions like acne, psoriasis, and eczema. An anti-inflammatory diet rich in antioxidants, vitamins, and healthy fats can promote clear, healthy skin. Foods like avocados, berries, and green tea provide essential nutrients that help reduce skin inflammation and enhance overall skin appearance.

6. Enhanced Immune Function

A strong immune system is supported by a nutritious, balanced diet. Anti-inflammatory foods such as garlic, ginger, and citrus fruits contain vitamins and minerals that boost immune function and help the body fight off infections more effectively. By reducing inflammation, the immune system can operate more efficiently without being overactive or compromised.

7. Weight Management

Inflammation can interfere with the body's ability to regulate metabolism, often leading to weight gain and obesity. An anti-inflammatory diet, emphasizing whole foods and healthy fats, can help maintain a healthy weight. High-fiber foods keep you feeling full longer, reducing the likelihood of overeating and promoting sustainable weight loss.

8. Increased Energy Levels

Chronic inflammation can sap your energy, leaving you feeling fatigued and sluggish.

By reducing inflammation, an anti-inflammatory diet can lead to increased energy levels. Nutrient-rich foods provide the essential vitamins and minerals your body needs to produce energy, keeping you feeling vibrant and active throughout the day.

9. Longevity

Age-related disorders and the aging process are both influenced by inflammation. By reducing chronic inflammation, you can improve your chances of living a longer, healthier life. The antioxidants in anti-inflammatory foods protect cells from damage, slowing down the aging process and promoting longevity.

10. Improved Quality of Life

Overall, adopting an anti-inflammatory diet can lead to a higher quality of life. With reduced pain, better mental health, increased energy, and a lower risk of chronic diseases, you can enjoy a more active and fulfilling life.

Basic Principles and Guidelines

Adopting an anti-inflammatory diet involves making mindful choices about the foods you eat and how you prepare them. By following these basic principles and guidelines, you can create a balanced and sustainable eating plan that supports your health and well-being.

1. Emphasize Whole, Unprocessed Foods

The foundation of an anti-inflammatory diet is whole, minimally processed foods. These foods are packed with nutrients and free from the additives and preservatives found in many processed items. Focus on:

Fruits and veggies: Try to include a range of vibrant fruits and veggies to fill half of your plate.

They are rich in antioxidants, vitamins, and minerals that help combat inflammation.

Whole Grains: Refined grains should be avoided in favor of whole grains including brown rice, quinoa, oats, and whole wheat. They provide fiber and nutrients that support digestive health and reduce inflammation.

Lean Proteins: Incorporate sources of lean protein such as poultry, fish, beans, lentils, and tofu. These provide essential amino acids without the inflammatory effects of processed meats.

Healthy Fats:Add foods like avocados, almonds, seeds, and olive oil that are good sources of fat. These fats are good for the heart and contain anti-inflammatory qualities.

2. Incorporate Anti-Inflammatory Foods

Certain foods have been shown to have powerful anti-inflammatory effects. Make sure to include these in your diet regularly:

Berries: Antioxidant-rich blueberries, strawberries, raspberries, and blackberries can help lower inflammation.

Leafy Greens: Spinach, kale, and Swiss chard are nutrient-dense and contain compounds that fight inflammation.

Fatty Fish: Salmon, mackerel, sardines, and trout are rich in omega-3 fatty acids, which are known for their anti-inflammatory benefits.

Nuts and Seeds: Nuts including flaxseeds, chia seeds, walnuts, and almonds are excellent providers of antioxidants and healthy fats.

Herbs and Spices: Turmeric, ginger, garlic, and cinnamon have potent anti-inflammatory properties and can enhance the flavor of your meals.

3. Limit Pro-Inflammatory Foods

Some foods can promote inflammation and should be consumed in moderation or avoided:

Processed Foods: Items high in refined sugars, trans fats, and artificial additives can increase inflammation. This includes snacks, sweets, fast food, and pre-packaged meals.

Refined Carbohydrates: White bread, pastries, and sugary cereals can cause spikes in blood sugar and contribute to inflammation.

Red and Processed Meats: Limit consumption of red meat and processed meats like sausages and bacon, which have been linked to increased inflammation.

Sugary Beverages: Soft drinks, energy drinks, and excessive fruit juices can lead to inflammation due to their high sugar content.

4. Stay Hydrated

Proper hydration is essential for overall health and can help reduce inflammation. Make it a point to stay hydrated during the day. Herbal teas and water-infused with fruits and herbs are also good options.

5. Practice Balanced Eating

Portion Control: Be mindful of portion sizes to avoid overeating, which can lead to weight gain and increased inflammation.

Balanced Meals: Strive for balance in each meal by including a mix of proteins, fats, and carbohydrates. This gives long-lasting energy and aids in maintaining stable blood sugar levels.

6. Prepare Meals Mindfully

Cooking Methods: Opt for cooking methods that preserve nutrients and minimize the formation of inflammatory compounds. Steaming, baking, grilling, and sautéing are preferable to frying.

Herbs and Spices: Use fresh or dried herbs and spices to flavor your dishes instead of relying on salt and sugar-laden sauces and condiments.

7. Lifestyle Factors

Regular Exercise: Incorporate regular physical activity into your routine. Exercise promotes general health and lowers inflammation.

Stress Management: Practice stress-reducing activities such as meditation, yoga, deep breathing, and spending time in nature. Chronic stress can contribute to inflammation.

Adequate Sleep: Make sure you get plenty of good sleep every night. Poor sleep can increase inflammation and negatively impact health.

Chapter 2: Stocking your Anti-inflammatory Pantry

Essential Ingredients

An anti-inflammatory diet focuses on incorporating ingredients that help reduce inflammation and support overall health. Here's a guide to some of the essential ingredients you should include in your pantry and refrigerator to create a balanced and effective anti-inflammatory diet:

1. Fruits

Berries: Blueberries, strawberries, raspberries, and blackberries are rich in antioxidants and vitamins that help combat inflammation.

Citrus Fruits: Oranges, lemons, limes, and grapefruits are high in vitamin C and antioxidants that support immune function and reduce inflammation.

Avocados: Packed with healthy fats, fiber, and antioxidants, avocados help reduce inflammation and promote heart health.

2. Vegetables

Leafy Greens: Spinach, kale, Swiss chard, and arugula are loaded with vitamins, minerals, and antioxidants that help fight inflammation.

Cruciferous Vegetables: Broccoli, Brussels sprouts, cauliflower, and cabbage contain compounds that support the body's detoxification processes and reduce inflammation.

Bell Peppers: Rich in vitamins A and C, as well as antioxidants, bell peppers can help lower inflammation.

3. Whole Grains

Quinoa: A complete protein and rich in fiber, quinoa is a great alternative to refined grains.

Brown Rice: Provides fiber and essential nutrients without the inflammatory effects of white rice.

Oats: Contain beta-glucan, a type of soluble fiber that helps reduce inflammation and supports heart health.

4. Healthy Fats

Olive Oil: Extra virgin olive oil is high in monounsaturated fats and antioxidants, which have anti-inflammatory properties.

Nuts: Almonds, walnuts, and Brazil nuts are rich in healthy fats, vitamins, and minerals that support anti-inflammatory processes.

Seeds: Flaxseeds, chia seeds, and hemp seeds are excellent sources of omega-3 fatty acids and fiber.

5. Lean Proteins

Fatty Fish: Salmon, mackerel, sardines, and trout are high in omega-3 fatty acids, which are known for their anti-inflammatory effects.

Poultry: Chicken and turkey provide lean protein without the inflammatory effects of red meats.

Legumes: Beans, lentils, and chickpeas are great plant-based protein sources that also provide fiber and essential nutrients.

6. Herbs and Spices

Turmeric: includes curcumin, an ingredient with potent antioxidant and anti-inflammatory qualities.

Ginger: Known for its ability to reduce inflammation and aid digestion.

Garlic: Has anti-inflammatory and immune-boosting effects, and can add flavor to dishes without extra salt or sugar.

Cinnamon: Provides antioxidants and can help regulate blood sugar levels.

7. Dairy Alternatives

Almond Milk: A dairy-free alternative rich in vitamins and low in inflammation-promoting additives.

Coconut Yogurt: A non-dairy yogurt option that can be rich in probiotics and free from inflammatory dairy proteins.

8. Beverages

Green Tea: Contains antioxidants such as catechins that help reduce inflammation.

Herbal Teas: Chamomile, peppermint, and rooibos teas offer anti-inflammatory and soothing properties.

9. Condiments and Sauces

Apple Cider Vinegar: Helps balance blood sugar levels and supports digestion.

Tamari: A gluten-free soy sauce alternative that can add umami flavor without inflammatory additives found in regular soy sauce.

10. Sweeteners

Raw Honey: A natural sweetener with anti-inflammatory and antioxidant properties.

Maple Syrup: Contains antioxidants and can be used in moderation as a healthier sweetening option compared to refined sugars.

Herbs and Spices for Reducing Inflammation

Incorporating herbs and spices into your diet can significantly reduce inflammation and enhance your overall health. Many herbs and spices contain powerful anti-inflammatory compounds that help combat chronic inflammation, support immune function, and provide additional health benefits. Here's a list of some of the most effective herbs and spices for reducing inflammation:

1. Turmeric
Key Compound: Curcumin
Benefits: Curcumin is a potent anti-inflammatory and antioxidant that helps neutralize free radicals and reduce inflammation. It has been shown to be effective in managing conditions like arthritis and inflammatory bowel disease.
How to Use: Add turmeric to curries, soups, stews, or smoothies. Consider combining it with black pepper for maximum absorption.

2. Ginger
Key Compound: Gingerol
Benefits: Gingerol has strong anti-inflammatory properties and can help alleviate symptoms of osteoarthritis and muscle pain. Ginger also aids digestion and can reduce nausea.
How to Use: Use fresh ginger in teas, stir-fries, and marinades, or add ground ginger to smoothies and baked goods.

3. Garlic
Key Compound: Allicin
Benefits: Allicin has anti-inflammatory, antioxidant, and antimicrobial properties.

Garlic can help reduce the risk of heart disease and support immune health.

How to Use: Incorporate minced or crushed garlic into savory dishes, soups, and salad dressings.

4. Cinnamon

Key Compound: Cinnamaldehyde

Benefits: Cinnamaldehyde has anti-inflammatory effects and can help regulate blood sugar levels. Cinnamon also contains antioxidants that support overall health.

How to Use: Sprinkle cinnamon on oatmeal, yogurt, smoothies, or baked goods.

5. Rosemary

Key Compound: Carnosol and rosmarinic acid

Benefits: Rosemary has antioxidant and anti-inflammatory properties that can help reduce oxidative stress and inflammation. It also supports cognitive function and digestion.

How to Use: Use fresh or dried rosemary in roasted vegetables, meats, and Mediterranean dishes.

6. Thyme

Key Compound: Thymol

Benefits: Thymol has anti-inflammatory and antimicrobial effects. Thyme can help soothe respiratory issues and support overall immune health.

How to Use: Add fresh or dried thyme to soups, stews, and marinades.

7. Oregano

Key Compound: Carvacrol

Benefits: Carvacrol has strong anti-inflammatory and antioxidant properties. Oregano can support digestive health and help fight off infections.

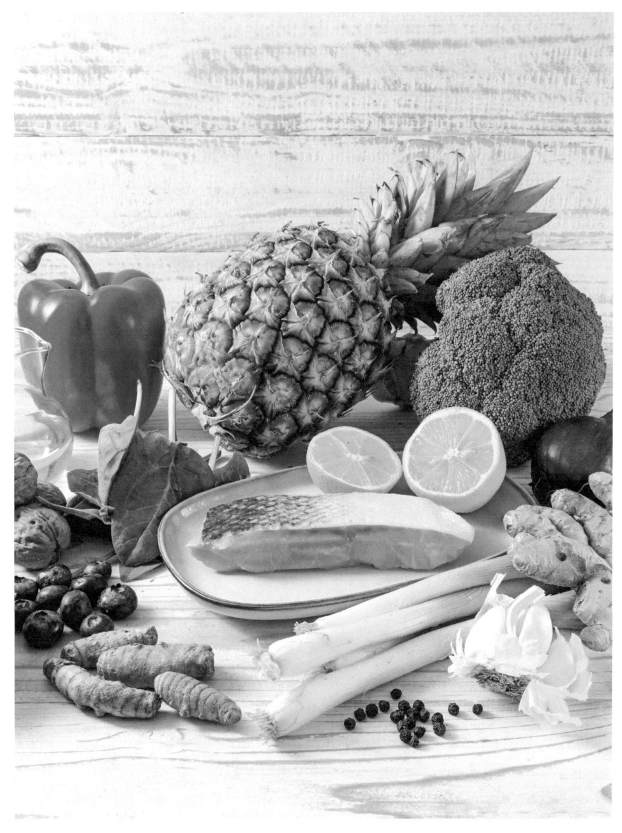

How to Use: Use oregano in Italian dishes, sauces, and as a seasoning for meats and vegetables.

8. Cloves
Key Compound: Eugenol

Benefits: Eugenol has powerful anti-inflammatory and antioxidant properties. Cloves can also help improve digestive health and reduce pain.

How to Use: Use ground cloves in baking, spice blends, and savory dishes, or steep whole cloves in teas.

9. Cayenne Pepper
Key Compound: Capsaicin

Benefits: Capsaicin has anti-inflammatory and pain-relieving properties. It can help reduce symptoms of arthritis and improve circulation.

How to Use: Add cayenne pepper to soups, stews, and spice blends for a kick of heat.

10. Fennel Seeds
Key Compound: Anethole

Benefits: Anethole has anti-inflammatory and antioxidant effects. Fennel seeds can aid digestion and reduce bloating.

How to Use: Chew fennel seeds after meals, or use them in spice blends and teas.

11. Holy Basil (Tulsi)
Key Compound: Ursolic acid

Benefits: Holy basil has anti-inflammatory, adaptogenic, and antioxidant properties. It can help manage stress and support overall well-being.

How to Use: Brew holy basil leaves into tea or use it in soups and stews.

12. Dandelion

Key Compound: Taraxasterol

Benefits: Dandelion has anti-inflammatory and diuretic properties. It supports liver health and can help reduce inflammation in the body.

How to Use: Use dandelion leaves in salads or brew them into a tea.

Grocery Shopping Tips

Grocery shopping for an anti-inflammatory diet can be straightforward and rewarding if you follow a few key tips. Focusing on whole, nutrient-dense foods and avoiding items that promote inflammation will help you build a healthy, balanced diet. Here's how to make the most of your grocery shopping experience:

1. Plan Your Meals

Establish a Weekly Menu: Arrange your meals for the coming week. This helps you determine what ingredients you need and prevents impulse buys.

Make a Shopping List: Based on your meal plan, write down a list of items you need. Stick to this list to avoid purchasing unnecessary or inflammatory foods.

2. Stick to the Perimeter

Shop the Outer Aisles: The perimeter of most grocery stores typically houses fresh produce, dairy, meat, and seafood. These areas generally contain less processed foods compared to the inner aisles.

Avoid Processed Foods: The inner aisles often contain packaged and processed foods high in sugars, unhealthy fats, and additives. Don't spend too much time in these places.

4. Select Whole Grains

Read Labels: Choose whole grains like brown rice, quinoa, and whole wheat. Look for products labeled "100% whole grain" and check the ingredient list to ensure whole grains are the first ingredient.

Avoid Refined Grains: Steer clear of products containing refined grains or added sugars, such as white bread and sugary cereals.

5. Choose Healthy Fats

Opt for Fresh Nuts and Seeds: Buy raw or lightly roasted nuts and seeds, such as almonds, walnuts, flaxseeds, and chia seeds.

Look for High-Quality Oils: Choose extra virgin olive oil, avocado oil, and coconut oil for cooking and dressings. Avoid oils high in trans fats, like vegetable oils and margarine.

6. Select Lean Proteins

Buy Fresh or Frozen Fish: Opt for wild-caught fish like salmon, mackerel, and sardines, which are high in anti-inflammatory omega-3 fatty acids.

Choose Lean Cuts of Meat: Look for lean poultry options like chicken and turkey. Steer clear of processed meats like bacon and sausages.

Stock Up on Legumes: Beans, lentils, and chickpeas are excellent plant-based protein sources. Buy them dried or canned (without added sodium).

7. Incorporate Herbs and Spices

Fresh and Dried: Buy fresh herbs like basil, cilantro, and parsley when available. For dried herbs and spices, select high-quality options without added salt or sugars.

Explore New Varieties: Experiment with different anti-inflammatory spices such as turmeric, ginger, and cinnamon to add flavor and health benefits to your meals.

8. Be Mindful of Beverages

Choose Herbal Teas: Look for options like green tea, chamomile, or ginger tea, which have anti-inflammatory properties.

Avoid Sugary Drinks: Skip sodas, energy drinks, and sugary fruit juices. Instead, opt for water, herbal teas, and sparkling water with a splash of lemon or lime.

9. Check Ingredient Lists

Watch for Hidden Sugars and Additives: Read ingredient labels carefully to avoid hidden sugars, trans fats, and artificial additives. Look for items with short ingredient lists and recognizable ingredients.

Choose Whole Foods: Whenever possible, select items with minimal or no processing.

10. Buy in Bulk

Non-Perishables: Purchasing items like grains, nuts, seeds, and dried beans in bulk can be cost-effective and reduce trips to the store.

Frozen Produce: Frozen fruits and vegetables can be a convenient and budget-friendly option while retaining their nutritional value.

11. Store Properly

Preserve Freshness: Store fruits and vegetables properly to maintain their freshness. Use airtight containers for nuts and seeds to prevent spoilage.

Plan for Leftovers: Prepare larger batches of meals and store leftovers in the freezer to have healthy options readily available.

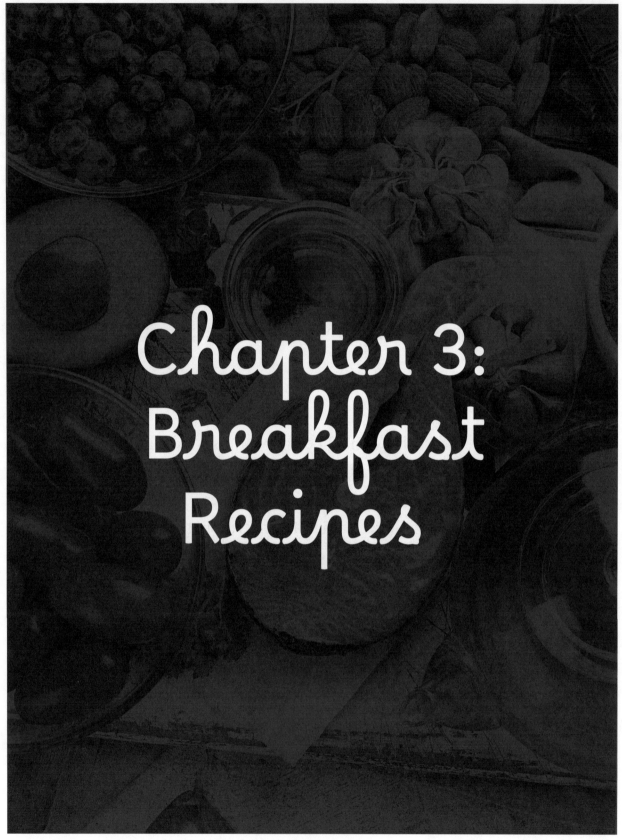

Chapter 3:
Breakfast
Recipes

Berry Chia Pudding

Prep 10 mim

Serves : 2

Cook None

Easy

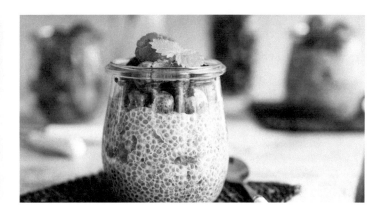

COOKING STEPS

1. In a bowl, mix chia seeds, almond milk, maple syrup, and vanilla extract.
2. Stir well, cover, and refrigerate for at least 4 hours or overnight.
3. Before serving, stir the pudding again and top with mixed berries.

INGREDIENTS

- 1/4 cup chia seeds
- 1 cup almond milk (or any non-dairy milk)
- 1 tablespoon maple syrup (or raw honey)
- 1/2 teaspoon vanilla extract
- 1/2 cup mixed berries (blueberries, strawberries, raspberries)

- Calories: 230, Protein: 6g, Carbohydrates: 30g, Fiber: 11g, Fat: 10g, Sugars: 8g

Avocado Toast with Turkey and Spinach

Prep 10 mim

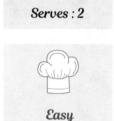
Serves : 2

Cook : 5 min

Easy

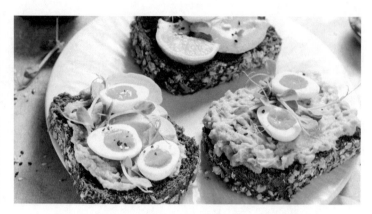

COOKING STEPS

1. Toast the whole-grain bread slices.
2. Mash the avocado in a bowl and season with salt and pepper.
3. Spread mashed avocado on toasted bread.
4. Top with turkey slices, fresh spinach, and a drizzle of olive oil.
5. Sprinkle with red pepper flakes if desired.

INGREDIENTS

- 1 ripe avocado
- 2 slices of whole-grain bread
- 4 slices of turkey breast (low sodium)
- 1 cup fresh spinach
- 1 tablespoon olive oil
- Salt and pepper to taste
- Red pepper flakes (optional)

- Calories: 320, Protein: 22g, Carbohydrates: 34g, Fiber: 9g, Fat: 14g, Sugars: 4g

Green Smoothie Bowl

Prep 10 mim

Serves : 1

Cook None

Easy

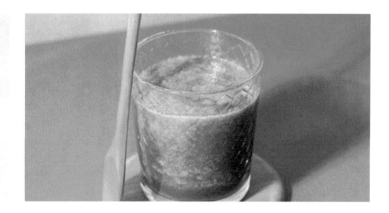

COOKING STEPS

1. In a blender, combine spinach, banana, mango, almond milk, and chia seeds.
2. Blend until smooth and creamy.
3. Pour the smoothie into a bowl and top with almond butter, granola, and sliced almonds.

INGREDIENTS

- 1 cup spinach leaves
- 1 banana
- 1/2 cup frozen mango chunks
- 1/2 cup almond milk (or any non-dairy milk)
- 1 tablespoon chia seeds
- 1 tablespoon almond butter
- 1/4 cup granola
- 1/4 cup sliced almonds

- Calories: 230, Protein: 6g, Carbohydrates: 30g, Fiber: 11g, Fat: 10g, Sugars: 8g

Sweet Potato and Black Bean Breakfast Burrito

Prep 10 mim

Serves : 1

Cook: 15 min

Easy

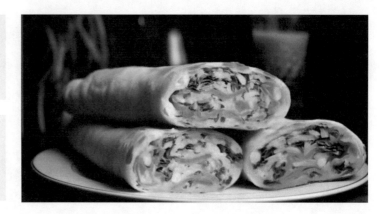

COOKING STEPS

1. Heat olive oil in a skillet over medium heat.
2. Add sweet potato and cook until tender, about 10 minutes.
3. Stir in black beans, cumin, paprika, and garlic powder; cook for another 2 minutes.
4. Warm tortillas in a separate pan or microwave.
5. Divide the sweet potato mixture between tortillas and top with salsa.
6. Roll up the tortillas and serve.

INGREDIENTS

- 1 medium sweet potato, peeled and diced
- 1/2 cup canned black beans, drained and rinsed
- 1 tablespoon olive oil
- 1/2 teaspoon cumin
- 1/2 teaspoon paprika
- 1/4 teaspoon garlic powder
- 2 whole-grain tortillas
- 1/4 cup salsa

- Calories: 350, Protein: 10g, Carbohydrates: 55g, Fiber: 10g, Fat: 12g, Sugars: 8g

Overnight Oats with Almonds and Berries

Prep : 5 min

Serves : 2

Cook : None

Easy

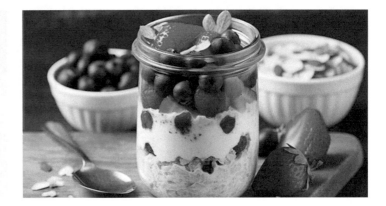

COOKING STEPS

1. Heat olive oil in a skillet over medium heat.
2. Add sweet potato and cook until tender, about 10 minutes.
3. Stir in black beans, cumin, paprika, and garlic powder; cook for another 2 minutes.
4. Warm tortillas in a separate pan or microwave.
5. Divide the sweet potato mixture between tortillas and top with salsa.
6. Roll up the tortillas and serve.In a jar or bowl, combine oats, almond milk, chia seeds, and maple syrup.
7. Stir well, cover, and refrigerate overnight.
8. Before serving, stir the oats and top with chopped almonds and mixed berries.

INGREDIENTS

- 1/2 cup rolled oats
- 1/2 cup almond milk (or any non-dairy milk)
- 1/4 cup chopped almonds
- 1 tablespoon chia seeds
- 1 tablespoon maple syrup (or raw honey)
- 1/2 cup mixed berries (blueberries, strawberries, raspberries)

- Calories: 300, Protein: 8g, Carbohydrates: 40g, Fiber: 10g, Fat: 14g, Sugars: 10g

Quinoa Breakfast Bowl with Veggies

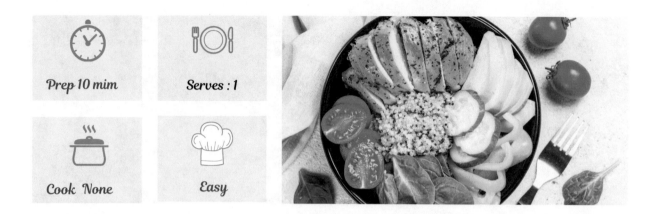

Prep 10 mim

Serves : 1

Cook None

Easy

COOKING STEPS

1. In a bowl, combine cooked quinoa, cherry tomatoes, avocado, and cucumber.
2. Drizzle with olive oil and lemon juice.
3. Season with salt and pepper, and toss to combine.

INGREDIENTS

- 1/2 cup cooked quinoa
- 1/2 cup cherry tomatoes, halved
- 1/2 avocado, diced
- 1/4 cup cucumber, diced
- 1 tablespoon olive oil
- 1 tablespoon lemon juice
- Salt and pepper to taste

- Calories: 300, Protein: 8g, Carbohydrates: 35g, Fiber: 7g, Fat: 15g, Sugars: 5g

Greek Yogurt with Honey and Nuts

Prep 5 min

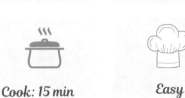

Serves : 1

Cook: 15 min

Easy

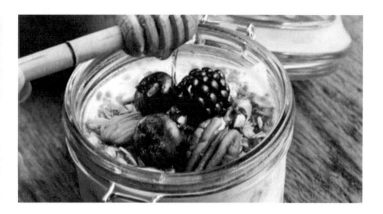

COOKING STEPS

1. Scoop Greek yogurt into a bowl.
2. Drizzle with raw honey.
3. Top with mixed nuts and chia seeds.

INGREDIENTS

- 1 cup plain Greek yogurt
- 1 tablespoon raw honey
- 2 tablespoons mixed nuts (almonds, walnuts, pecans)
- 1 tablespoon chia seeds

- Calories: 320, Protein: 20g, Carbohydrates: 30g, Fiber: 6g, Fat: 16g, Sugars: 15g

Spinach and Mushroom Frittata

Prep 10 mim

Serves : 2

Cook : 20 min

Easy

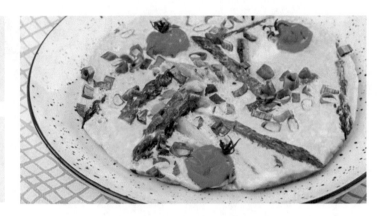

COOKING STEPS

1. Preheat the oven to 375°F (190°C).
2. Heat olive oil in a skillet over medium heat. Add mushrooms and cook until tender.
3. Add spinach and cook until wilted.
4. In a bowl, whisk eggs and season with salt and pepper
5. Pour eggs over the vegetables in the skillet. Sprinkle with feta cheese.
6. Transfer the skillet to the oven and bake for 15-20 minutes, until the eggs are set.

INGREDIENTS

- 4 large eggs
- 1 cup fresh spinach, chopped
- 1/2 cup mushrooms, sliced
- 1/4 cup feta cheese, crumbled
- 1 tablespoon olive oil
- Salt and pepper to taste

- Calories: 350, Protein: 10g, Carbohydrates: 55g, Fiber: 10g, Fat: 12g, Sugars: 8g

Almond Butter Banana Toast

Prep : 5 min

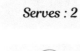

Serves : 2

Cook : 5 min

Easy

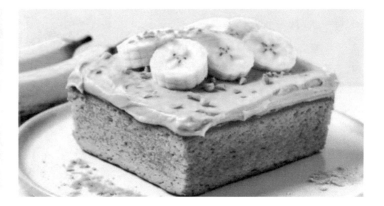

COOKING STEPS

1. Toast the whole-grain bread slices.
2. Spread almond butter evenly on the toasted bread.
3. Top with banana slices, chia seeds, and a sprinkle of cinnamon.

INGREDIENTS

- 1 banana, sliced
- 2 slices whole-grain bread
- 2 tablespoons almond butter
- 1 tablespoon chia seeds
- 1/2 teaspoon cinnamon

- Calories: 350, Protein: 10g, Carbohydrates: 45g, Fiber: 7g, Fat: 16g, Sugars: 15g

Apple Cinnamon Overnight Oats

Prep : 5 min

Serves : 1

Cook : None

Easy

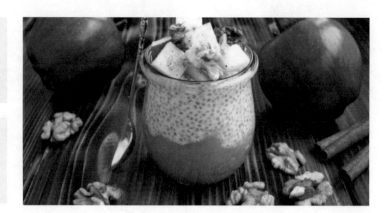

COOKING STEPS

1. In a jar or bowl, combine oats, almond milk, chia seeds, cinnamon, and maple syrup.
2. Stir well to mix all ingredients.
3. Add diced apple and mix again.
4. Cover and refrigerate overnight.
5. In the morning, stir the oats and enjoy as is or topped with additional apple slices and a sprinkle of cinnamon.

INGREDIENTS

- 1/2 cup rolled oats
- 1/2 cup almond milk (or any non-dairy milk)
- 1/2 apple, diced
- 1 tablespoon chia seeds
- 1/2 teaspoon cinnamon
- 1 tablespoon maple syrup (or raw honey)

- Calories: 300, Protein: 7g, Carbohydrates: 50g, Fiber: 8g, Fat: 8g, Sugars: 15g

Chapter 4:
Lunch Recipes

Quinoa Salad with Chickpeas and Avocado

Prep: 15 min

Serves : 2

Cook : None

Easy

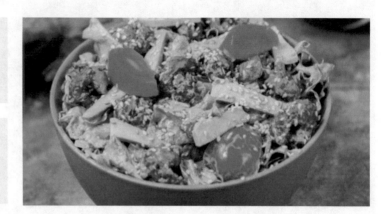

COOKING STEPS

1. In a large bowl, combine cooked quinoa, chickpeas, avocado, cherry tomatoes, red onion, and parsley.
2. In a small bowl, whisk together olive oil, lemon juice, salt, and pepper.
3. Pour the dressing over the salad and toss to combine.
4. Serve immediately or refrigerate for later.

INGREDIENTS

- 1 cup cooked quinoa
- 1 cup canned chickpeas, drained and rinsed
- 1 avocado, diced
- 1/2 cup cherry tomatoes, halved
- 1/4 cup red onion, finely chopped
- 2 tablespoons fresh parsley, chopped
- 2 tablespoons olive oil
- 1 tablespoon lemon juice
- Salt and pepper to taste

- Calories: 350, Protein: 10g, Carbohydrates: 40g, Fiber: 12g, Fat: 18g, Sugars: 3g

Mediterranean Chickpea Wraps

Prep: 10 min

Serves : 2

Cook : None

Easy

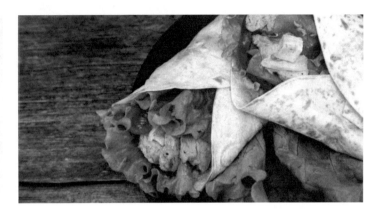

COOKING STEPS

1. In a bowl, combine chickpeas, cucumber, cherry tomatoes, red onion, feta cheese, olive oil, lemon juice, salt, and pepper.
2. Spread hummus evenly on each tortilla.
3. Divide the chickpea mixture between the tortillas.
4. Roll up the tortillas and serve.

INGREDIENTS

- 1 cup canned chickpeas, drained and rinsed
- 1/2 cup cucumber, diced
- 1/2 cup cherry tomatoes, halved
- 1/4 cup red onion, finely chopped
- 1/4 cup feta cheese, crumbled
- 2 tablespoons hummus
- 2 whole-grain tortillas
- 1 tablespoon olive oil
- 1 tablespoon lemon juice
- Salt and pepper to taste

- Calories: 350, Protein: 11g, Carbohydrates: 42g, Fiber: 9g, Fat: 15g, Sugars: 4g

Grilled Chicken and Vegetable Skewers

 Prep: 15 min

 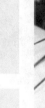 Serves : 2

 Cook: 12 mim

Easy

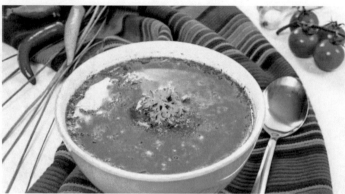

COOKING STEPS

1. Preheat the grill to medium-high heat.
2. In a bowl, combine olive oil, lemon juice, oregano, salt, and pepper.
3. Thread chicken and vegetables onto the skewers.
4. Brush the skewers with the olive oil mixture.
5. Grill for 10-12 minutes, turning occasionally, until the chicken is cooked through and vegetables are tender.
6. Serve with a side salad or whole-grain rice.

INGREDIENTS

- 2 boneless, skinless chicken breasts, cut into 1-inch cubes
- 1 red bell pepper, cut into 1-inch pieces
- 1 zucchini, cut into 1-inch pieces
- 1 red onion, cut into 1-inch pieces
- 2 tablespoons olive oil
- 1 tablespoon lemon juice
- 1 teaspoon dried oregano
- Salt and pepper to taste
- Wooden skewers, soaked in water for 30 minutes

- Calories: 300, Protein: 28g, Carbohydrates: 10g, Fiber: 3g, Fat: 16g, Sugars: 5g

Lentil and Vegetable Soup

Prep: 10 min

Serves : 4

Cook : 30 min

Easy

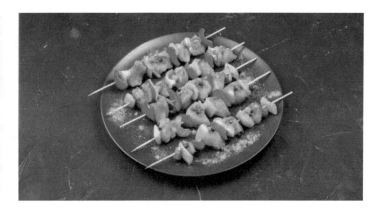

COOKING STEPS

1. In a large pot, heat olive oil over medium heat. Add onion, carrot, celery, and garlic; sauté until vegetables are tender.
2. Add lentils, diced tomatoes, vegetable broth, cumin, turmeric, salt, and pepper.
3. Bring to a boil, then reduce heat and simmer for 30 minutes, or until lentils are tender.
4. Serve hot.

INGREDIENTS

- 1 cup dry lentils, rinsed
- 1 carrot, diced
- 1 celery stalk, diced
- 1 onion, diced
- 2 garlic cloves, minced
- 1 can (14.5 ounces) diced tomatoes
- 4 cups vegetable broth
- 1 teaspoon ground cumin
- 1 teaspoon ground turmeric
- 2 tablespoons olive oil
- Salt and pepper to taste

- Calories: 250, Protein: 12g, Carbohydrates: 35g, Fiber: 15g, Fat: 6g, Sugars: 5g

Sweet Potato and Black Bean Tacos

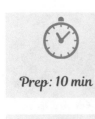
Prep: 10 min

Serves : 3

Cook : 25 min

Easy

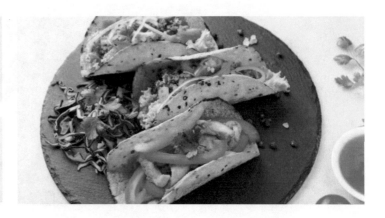

COOKING STEPS

1. Preheat the oven to 400°F (200°C).
2. In a bowl, toss sweet potato with olive oil, cumin, chili powder, garlic powder, salt, and pepper.
3. Spread sweet potato on a baking sheet and roast for 20-25 minutes, until tender.
4. Heat black beans in a small pot over medium heat.
5. Warm tortillas in a skillet or microwave.
6. Divide sweet potato and black beans between tortillas.
7. Top with avocado slices, cilantro, and a squeeze of lime.

INGREDIENTS

- 1 medium sweet potato, peeled and diced
- 1 can (15 ounces) black beans, drained and rinsed
- 1 tablespoon olive oil
- 1 teaspoon ground cumin
- 1 teaspoon chili powder
- 1/2 teaspoon garlic powder
- Salt and pepper to taste
- 6 small corn tortillas
- 1 avocado, sliced
- Fresh cilantro, chopped
- Lime wedges

- Calories: 300, Protein: 7g, Carbohydrates: 50g, Fiber: 8g, Fat: 8g, Sugars: 15g

Spinach and Quinoa Stuffed Bell Peppers

Prep : 15 min

Serves : 4

Cook: 35 min

Easy

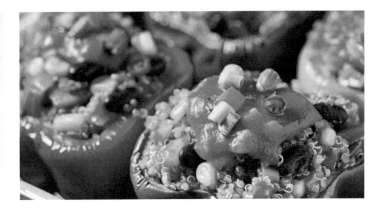

COOKING STEPS

1. Preheat the oven to 375°F (190°C).
2. In a large bowl, combine cooked quinoa, spinach, black beans, corn, red onion, olive oil, cumin, salt, and pepper.
3. Stuff each bell pepper with the quinoa mixture.
4. Place stuffed peppers in a baking dish and cover with foil.
5. Bake for 30 minutes.
6. If using cheese, remove foil, sprinkle cheese on top, and bake for an additional 5 minutes, until cheese is melted.
7. Serve hot.

- Calories: 300, Protein: 7g, Carbohydrates: 50g, Fiber: 8g, Fat: 8g, Sugars: 15g

INGREDIENTS

- 4 bell peppers, tops cut off and seeds removed
- 1 cup cooked quinoa
- 2 cups fresh spinach, chopped
- 1/2 cup canned black beans, drained and rinsed
- 1/2 cup corn kernels (fresh or frozen)
- 1/4 cup red onion, finely chopped
- 1 tablespoon olive oil
- 1 teaspoon cumin
- Salt and pepper to taste
- 1/4 cup shredded cheese (optional)

Grilled Salmon Salad

Prep: 10 min

Serves : 2

Cook: 10 min

Easy

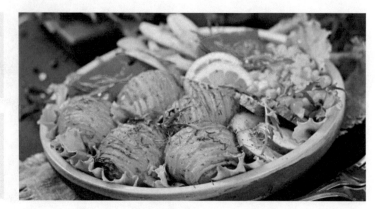

COOKING STEPS

1. Preheat the grill to medium-high heat.
2. Season salmon fillets with salt and pepper.
3. Grill salmon for 4-5 minutes per side, until cooked through.
4. In a large bowl, combine mixed greens, avocado, cherry tomatoes, and red onion.
5. In a small bowl, whisk together olive oil and lemon juice.
6. Drizzle the dressing over the salad and toss to combine.
7. Top the salad with grilled salmon.

INGREDIENTS

- 2 salmon fillets
- 4 cups mixed greens (spinach, arugula, kale)
- 1 avocado, sliced
- 1/2 cup cherry tomatoes, halved
- 1/4 cup red onion, thinly sliced
- 2 tablespoons olive oil
- 1 tablespoon lemon juice

- Calories: 450, Protein: 30g, Carbohydrates: 15g, Fiber: 7g, Fat: 32g, Sugars: 3g

Vegan Buddha Bowl

Prep: 10 min

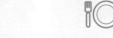
Serves : 1

Cook : None

Easy

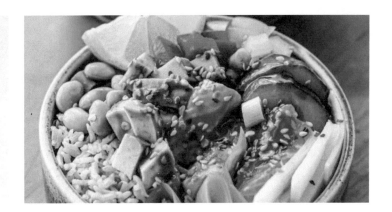

COOKING STEPS

1. In a bowl, arrange cooked brown rice, chickpeas, shredded carrots, avocado, and steamed broccoli.
2. In a small bowl, whisk together tahini, lemon juice, maple syrup, salt, and pepper.
3. Drizzle the tahini dressing over the bowl.
4. Serve immediately.

INGREDIENTS

- 1 cup cooked brown rice
- 1/2 cup chickpeas, drained and rinsed
- 1/2 cup shredded carrots
- 1/2 avocado, sliced
- 1/2 cup steamed broccoli
- 2 tablespoons tahini
- 1 tablespoon lemon juice
- 1 teaspoon maple syrup
- Salt and pepper to taste

- Calories: 450, Protein: 14g Carbohydrates: 60g, Fiber: 12g, Fat: 18g, Sugars: 7g

Turkey and Avocado Lettuce Wraps

Prep: 10 min

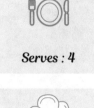
Serves : 4

Cook: 10 min

Easy

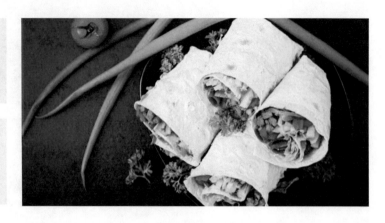

COOKING STEPS

1. In a skillet, heat olive oil over medium heat. Add ground turkey, smoked paprika, salt, and pepper. Cook until turkey is fully cooked.
2. To assemble wraps, place a few spoonfuls of cooked turkey onto each lettuce leaf.
3. Top with diced avocado, tomatoes, and red onion.
4. Serve immediately.

INGREDIENTS

- 8 large lettuce leaves (such as Romaine or Butter)
- 1 cup cooked ground turkey
- 1 avocado, diced
- 1/2 cup diced tomatoes
- 1/4 cup red onion, finely chopped
- 1 tablespoon olive oil
- 1 teaspoon smoked paprika
- Salt and pepper to taste

- Calories: 250, Protein: 20g, Carbohydrates: 12g, Fiber: 6g, Fat: 15g, Sugars: 3g

Cucumber and Hummus Sandwiches

Prep: 10 min

Serves : 2

Cook : None

Easy

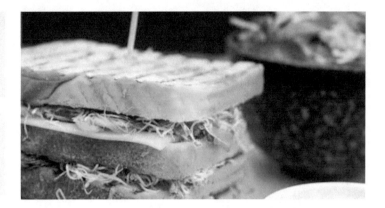

COOKING STEPS

1. Spread hummus evenly over each slice of bread.
2. Arrange cucumber slices on two of the bread slices.
3. Sprinkle with dill, lemon juice, salt, and pepper.
4. Top with the remaining bread slices to make sandwiches.
5. Cut into halves or quarters and serve.

INGREDIENTS

- 4 slices whole-grain bread
- 1/2 cup hummus
- 1 cucumber, thinly sliced
- 1/4 cup fresh dill, chopped
- 1 tablespoon lemon juice
- Salt and pepper to taste

- Calories: 300, Protein: 10g, Carbohydrates: 40g, Fiber: 8g, Fat: 12g, Sugars: 5g

Chapter 5: Dinner Recipes

Lemon Herb Baked Salmon

Prep: 10 min

Serves : 2

Cook: 15 min

Easy

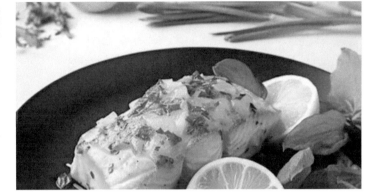

COOKING STEPS

1. Preheat the oven to 400°F (200°C).
2. Place the salmon fillets on a baking sheet lined with parchment paper.
3. In a small bowl, mix olive oil, lemon juice, thyme, rosemary, minced garlic, salt, and pepper.
4. Brush the mixture over the salmon fillets.
5. Bake for 12-15 minutes, until the salmon is cooked through and flakes easily with a fork.
6. Serve with a side of steamed vegetables or quinoa.

INGREDIENTS

- 2 salmon filets (6 oz each)
- 2 tablespoons olive oil
- 2 tablespoons lemon juice
- 1 teaspoon dried thyme
- 1 teaspoon dried rosemary
- 2 garlic cloves, minced
- Salt and pepper to taste

- Calories: 350, Protein: 30g, Carbohydrates: 3g, Fiber: 1g, Fat: 23g, Sugars: 0g

Stuffed Bell Peppers

Prep: 15 min

Serves : 4

Cook: 45 min

Easy

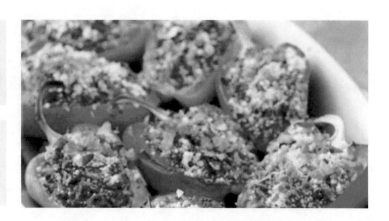

COOKING STEPS

1. In a bowl, mix cooked rice, ground turkey, black beans, corn, diced tomatoes, cumin, paprika, salt, and pepper.
2. Stuff each bell pepper with the mixture.
3. Place stuffed peppers in a baking dish and drizzle with olive oil.
4. Cover with foil and bake for 30 minutes.
5. Remove foil and bake for an additional 10 minutes until peppers are tender.

INGREDIENTS

- 4 bell peppers, tops cut off and seeds removed
- 1 cup cooked brown rice
- 1 cup cooked ground turkey
- 1/2 cup black beans, drained and rinsed
- 1/2 cup corn kernels
- 1/2 cup diced tomatoes
- 1 teaspoon ground cumin
- 1 teaspoon paprika
- 1 tablespoon olive oil
- Salt and pepper to taste

- Calories: 300, Protein: 20g, Carbohydrates: 40g, Fiber: 10g, Fat: 8g, Sugars: 8g

Sweet Potato and Black Bean Chili

Prep: 10 min

Serves : 4

Cook: 25 min

Easy

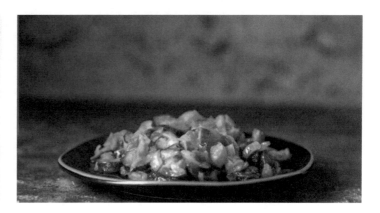

COOKING STEPS

1. In a large pot, heat olive oil over medium heat. Add onion and garlic, and sauté until translucent.
2. Add sweet potato and cook for 5 minutes.
3. Stir in black beans, diced tomatoes, vegetable broth, chili powder, cumin, salt, and pepper.
4. Bring to a boil, then reduce heat and simmer for 20-25 minutes, until sweet potatoes are tender.
5. Serve hot.

INGREDIENTS

- 1 tablespoon olive oil
- 1 onion, chopped
- 2 garlic cloves, minced
- 1 medium sweet potato, peeled and diced
- 1 can (15 oz) black beans, drained and rinsed
- 1 can (14.5 oz) diced tomatoes
- 1 cup vegetable broth
- 1 tablespoon chili powder
- 1 teaspoon cumin
- Salt and pepper to taste

- Calories: 250, Protein: 10g, Carbohydrates: 45g, Fiber: 12g, Fat: 7g, Sugars: 8g

Spinach and Feta Stuffed Chicken Breast

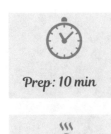
Prep: 10 min

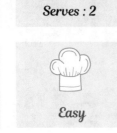
Serves : 2

Cook : 30 min

Easy

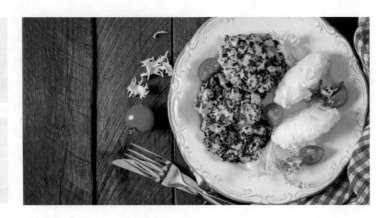

COOKING STEPS

1. Preheat the oven to 375°F (190°C).
2. Cut a pocket into each chicken breast.
3. In a bowl, mix spinach, feta cheese, salt, and pepper.
4. Stuff the mixture into the pockets of the chicken breasts.
5. Rub chicken breasts with olive oil and sprinkle with oregano.
6. Place chicken in a baking dish and bake for 25-30 minutes, until cooked through.

INGREDIENTS

- 2 boneless, skinless chicken breasts
- 1 cup fresh spinach, chopped
- 1/4 cup feta cheese, crumbled
- 1 tablespoon olive oil
- 1 teaspoon dried oregano
- Salt and pepper to taste

- Calories: 300, Protein: 30g, Carbohydrates: 3g, Fiber: 1g, Fat: 18g, Sugars: 1g

Zucchini Noodles with Avocado Pesto

Prep: 10 min

Serves : 2

Cook : None

Easy

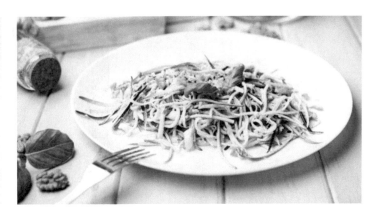

COOKING STEPS

1. In a food processor, combine avocado, basil, garlic, olive oil, lemon juice, salt, and pepper. Blend until smooth.
2. Toss zucchini noodles with the avocado pesto.
3. Serve immediately or chill before serving.

INGREDIENTS

- 2 large zucchinis, spiralized into noodles
- 1 avocado
- 1/2 cup fresh basil leaves
- 2 garlic cloves
- 2 tablespoons olive oil
- 1 tablespoon lemon juice
- Salt and pepper to taste

- Calories: 300, Protein: 4g, Carbohydrates: 16g, Fiber: 8g, Fat: 26g, Sugars: 4g

Cauliflower Rice Stir-Fry

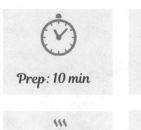

Prep: 10 min

Serves : 2

Cook: 10 min

Easy

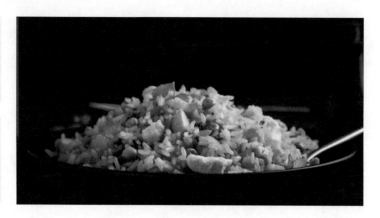

COOKING STEPS

1. Heat olive oil in a large skillet over medium heat.
2. Add garlic and ginger; cook for 1 minute.
3. Add mixed vegetables and cook for 5 minutes.
4. Stir in cauliflower rice and soy sauce; cook for another 5 minutes until cauliflower is tender.
5. Garnish with green onions and serve.

INGREDIENTS

- 1 head cauliflower, grated into rice-sized pieces
- 1 tablespoon olive oil
- 1 cup mixed vegetables (carrots, bell peppers, peas)
- 2 garlic cloves, minced
- 2 tablespoons low-sodium soy sauce or tamari
- 1 teaspoon grated ginger
- 2 green onions, chopped

- Calories: 200, Protein: 4g, Carbohydrates: 25g, Fiber: 7g, Fat: 10g, Sugars: 7g

Turmeric-Spiced Chicken and Veggies

Prep: 10 min

Serves : 2

Cook: 30 min

Easy

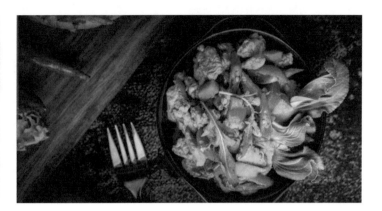

COOKING STEPS

1. Preheat the oven to 400°F (200°C).
2. In a bowl, toss chicken thighs, broccoli, and butternut squash with olive oil, turmeric, garlic powder, salt, and pepper.
3. Spread the mixture on a baking sheet.
4. Bake for 25-30 minutes, until chicken is cooked through and vegetables are tender.

INGREDIENTS

- 2 boneless, skinless chicken thighs
- 1 cup broccoli florets
- 1 cup diced butternut squash
- 2 tablespoons olive oil
- 1 teaspoon ground turmeric
- 1 teaspoon garlic powder
- Salt and pepper to taste

- Calories: 350, Protein: 25g,.Carbohydrates: 30g, Fiber: 8g, Fat: 18g, Sugars: 6g

Lentil and Kale Stew

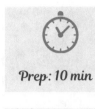 Prep: 10 min

 Serves : 4

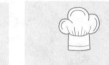 Cook: 30 min

Easy

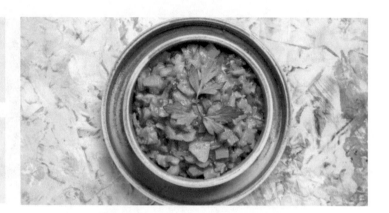

COOKING STEPS

1. Heat olive oil in a large pot over medium heat. Add onion and garlic; sauté until translucent.
2. Stir in lentils, kale, diced tomatoes, vegetable broth, paprika, thyme, salt, and pepper.
3. Bring to a boil, then reduce heat and simmer for 30 minutes, until lentils are tender.
4. Serve hot.

INGREDIENTS

- 1 tablespoon olive oil
- 1 onion, diced
- 2 garlic cloves, minced
- 1 cup dry lentils, rinsed
- 1 cup chopped kale
- 1 can (14.5 oz) diced tomatoes
- 4 cups vegetable broth
- 1 teaspoon paprika
- 1 teaspoon dried thyme
- Salt and pepper to taste

- Calories: 250, Protein: 12g, Carbohydrates: 40g, Fiber: 15g, Fat: 6g, Sugars: 7g

Baked Cod with Sweet Potatoes

Prep: 10 min

Serves : 2

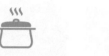

Cook: 35 min

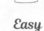

Easy

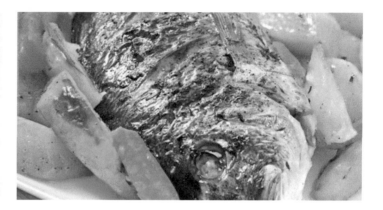

COOKING STEPS

1. Preheat the oven to 400°F (200°C).
2. Toss sweet potato cubes with 1 tablespoon of olive oil, paprika, garlic powder, salt, and pepper. Spread on a baking sheet.
3. Bake for 20 minutes.
4. Rub cod fillets with the remaining olive oil, salt, and pepper.
5. Place cod on the baking sheet with sweet potatoes and bake for an additional 15-20 minutes, until the cod is cooked through.
6. Serve with lemon wedges.

INGREDIENTS

- 2 cod filets (6 oz each)
- 2 medium sweet potatoes, peeled and diced
- 2 tablespoons olive oil
- 1 teaspoon paprika
- 1 teaspoon garlic powder
- Salt and pepper to taste
- Lemon wedges for serving

- Calories: 350, Protein: 30g, Carbohydrates: 30g, Fiber: 5g, Fat: 15g, Sugars: 8g

Garlic Shrimp and Asparagus

Prep: 10 min

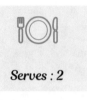
Serves : 2

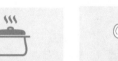
Cook: 10 min

Easy

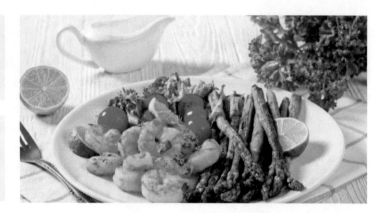

COOKING STEPS

1. Heat olive oil in a large skillet over medium heat.
2. Add garlic and red pepper flakes (if using); cook for 1 minute.
3. Add shrimp and cook for 3-4 minutes, until pink and opaque.
4. Add asparagus and cook for an additional 5 minutes, until tender-crisp.
5. Stir in lemon juice, salt, and pepper.
6. Serve immediately.

INGREDIENTS

- 1 pound large shrimp, peeled and deveined
- 1 bunch asparagus, trimmed and cut into 2-inch pieces
- 2 tablespoons olive oil
- 3 garlic cloves, minced
- 1/4 teaspoon red pepper flakes (optional)
- 1 tablespoon lemon juice
- Salt and pepper to taste

- Calories: 300, Protein: 30g, Carbohydrates: 10g, Fiber: 4g, Fat: 15g, Sugars: 4g

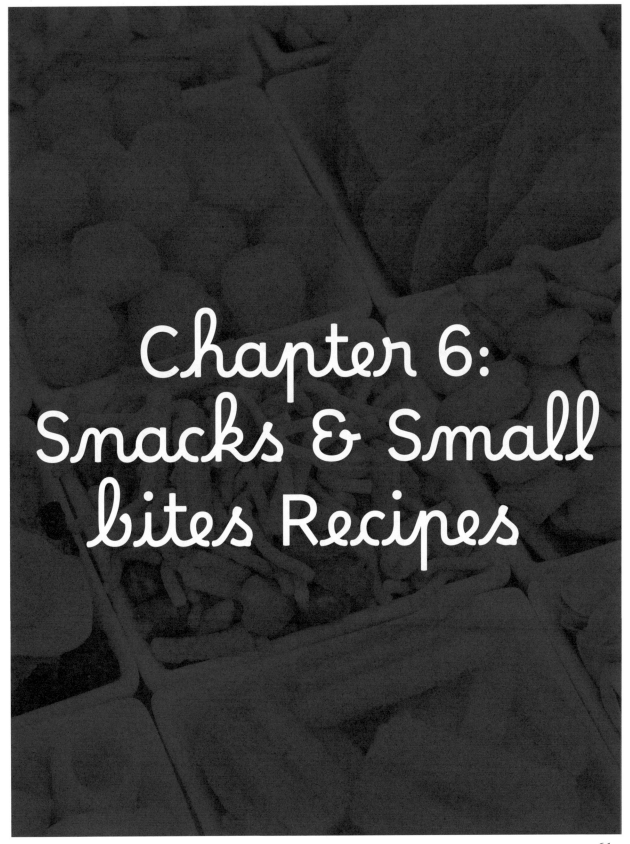

Chapter 6: Snacks & Small bites Recipes

Turmeric Roasted Chickpeas

Prep: 10 min

Serves : 4

Cook: 30 min

Easy

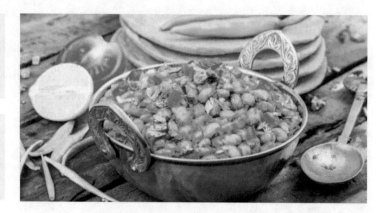

COOKING STEPS

1. Preheat the oven to 400°F (200°C).
2. Pat chickpeas dry with a paper towel.
3. In a bowl, toss chickpeas with olive oil, turmeric, paprika, garlic powder, and salt.
4. Spread chickpeas in a single layer on a baking sheet.
5. Roast for 25-30 minutes, shaking the pan halfway through, until chickpeas are crispy.
6. Let cool before serving.

INGREDIENTS

- 1 can (15 oz) chickpeas, drained and rinsed
- 1 tablespoon olive oil
- 1 teaspoon ground turmeric
- 1/2 teaspoon paprika
- 1/2 teaspoon garlic powder
- Salt to taste

- Calories: 150, Protein: 6g, Carbohydrates: 20g, Fiber: 6g, Fat: 6g, Sugars: 2g

Cucumber and Hummus Bites

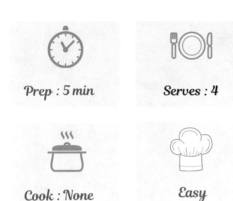

Prep : 5 min

Serves : 4

Cook : None

Easy

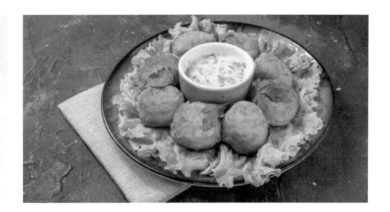

COOKING STEPS

1. Arrange cucumber slices on a serving platter.
2. Top each slice with a dollop of hummus.
3. Sprinkle with fresh dill, salt, and pepper.
4. Serve immediately.

INGREDIENTS

- 1 large cucumber, sliced into rounds
- 1/2 cup hummus
- 1 tablespoon fresh dill, chopped
- Salt and pepper to taste

- Calories: 100, Protein: 4g, Carbohydrates: 10g, Fiber: 3g, Fat: 6g, Sugars: 2g

Avocado and Tomato Salsa

 Prep: 10 min

 Serves : 4

 Cook : None

 Easy

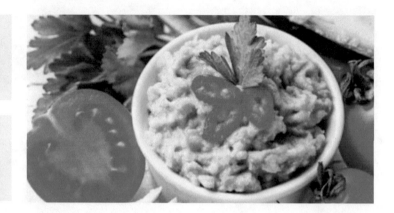

COOKING STEPS

1. In a bowl, combine avocado, cherry tomatoes, red onion, cilantro, and lime juice.
2. Season with salt and pepper.
3. Stir gently to combine.
4. Serve with whole-grain crackers or as a dip with vegetables.

INGREDIENTS

- 1 ripe avocado, diced
- 1 cup cherry tomatoes, halved
- 1/4 cup red onion, finely chopped
- 1 tablespoon fresh cilantro, chopped
- 1 tablespoon lime juice
- Salt and pepper to taste

- Calories: 180, Protein: 3g, Carbohydrates: 20g, Fiber: 7g, Fat: 10g, Sugars: 3g

Almond Butter Energy Balls

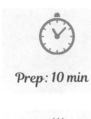

Prep: 10 min

Serves : 12

Cook : None

Easy

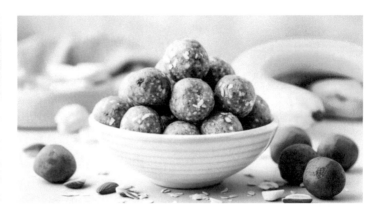

COOKING STEPS

1. In a bowl, mix together oats, almond butter, honey, chia seeds, and chocolate chips if using.
2. Roll mixture into 1-inch balls and place on a parchment-lined tray.
3. Refrigerate for at least 30 minutes to firm up.
4. Store in an airtight container in the fridge.

INGREDIENTS

- 1 cup rolled oats
- 1/2 cup almond butter
- 1/4 cup honey or maple syrup
- 1/4 cup chia seeds
- 1/4 cup dark chocolate chips (optional)

- Calories: 150, Protein: 5g, Carbohydrates: 18g, Fiber: 4g, Fat: 8g, Sugars: 8g

Greek Yogurt and Berry Parfait

 Prep : 5 min

 Serves : 2

 Cook : None

 Easy

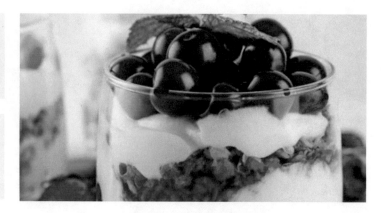

COOKING STEPS

1. In a serving glass or bowl, layer Greek yogurt, mixed berries, and granola if using.
2. Drizzle with honey or maple syrup.
3. Serve immediately.

INGREDIENTS

- 1 cup plain Greek yogurt
- 1/2 cup mixed berries (blueberries, strawberries, raspberries)
- 2 tablespoons granola (optional)
- 1 tablespoon honey or maple syrup

- Calories: 200, Protein: 12g, Carbohydrates: 30g, Fiber: 5g, Fat: 5g, Sugars: 15g

Roasted Red Pepper and Walnut Dip

Prep: 10 min

Serves : 4

Cook : None

Easy

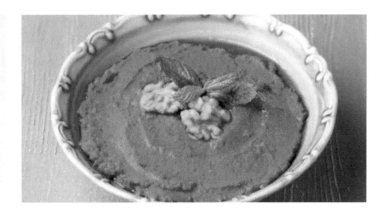

COOKING STEPS

1. In a food processor, combine roasted red peppers, walnuts, garlic, olive oil, lemon juice, salt, and pepper.
2. Process until smooth.
3. Serve with sliced vegetables or whole-grain pita chips.

INGREDIENTS

- 1 cup roasted red peppers (jarred or homemade)
- 1/2 cup walnuts
- 2 garlic cloves
- 2 tablespoons olive oil
- 1 tablespoon lemon juice
- Salt and pepper to taste

- Calories: 150, Protein: 4g, Carbohydrates: 10g, Fiber: 3g, Fat: 10g, Sugars: 3g

Apple Slices with Almond Butter

 Prep : 5 min

 Serves : 2

 Cook : None

 Easy

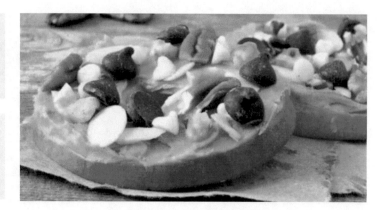

COOKING STEPS

1. Arrange apple slices on a plate.
2. Serve with a side of almond butter for dipping.
3. Sprinkle with chia seeds and cinnamon if desired.

INGREDIENTS

- 1 large apple, sliced
- 1/4 cup almond butter
- 1 tablespoon chia seeds (optional)
- Cinnamon for sprinkling (optional)

- Calories: 200, Protein: 4g, Carbohydrates: 25g, Fiber: 5g, Fat: 10g, Sugars: 15g

Carrot and Celery Sticks with Guacamole

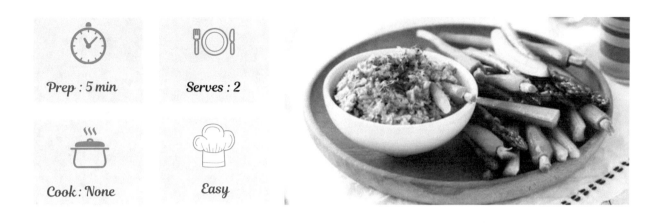

Prep : 5 min

Serves : 2

Cook : None

Easy

COOKING STEPS

1. Arrange carrot and celery sticks on a platter.
2. Serve with a bowl of guacamole for dipping.

INGREDIENTS

- 2 large carrots, peeled and cut into sticks
- 2 celery stalks, cut into sticks
- 1 cup guacamole

- Calories: 180, Protein: 3g, Carbohydrates: 20g, Fiber: 7g, Fat: 10g, Sugars: 5g

Baked Apple Chips

Prep: 10 min

Serves : 4

Cook 1.5 hrs

Easy

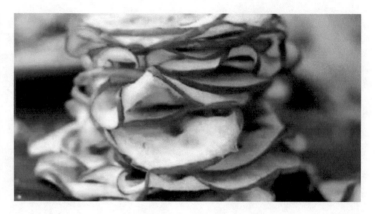

COOKING STEPS

1. Preheat the oven to 225°F (110°C).
2. Arrange apple slices in a single layer on a baking sheet.
3. Sprinkle it with cinnamon and nutmeg.
4. Bake for 1-1.5 hours, flipping halfway through, until apple slices are crispy.
5. Cool before serving.

INGREDIENTS

- 2 large apples, thinly sliced
- 1 teaspoon cinnamon
- 1/2 teaspoon nutmeg

- Calories: 100, Protein: 0g, Carbohydrates: 25g, Fiber: 5g, Fat: 0g, Sugars: 20g

Edamame with Sea Salt

Prep : 5 min

Serves : 4

Cook : 5 min

Easy

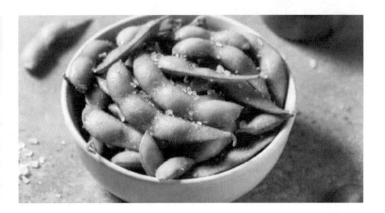

COOKING STEPS

1. Cook edamame according to package instructions (boil or steam).
2. Drain and toss with olive oil and sea salt.
3. Serve warm or at room temperature.

INGREDIENTS

- 2 cups shelled edamame (frozen or fresh)
- 1 tablespoon olive oil
- 1/2 teaspoon sea salt

- Calories: 150, Protein: 11g, Carbohydrates: 15g, Fiber: 6g, Fat: 7g, Sugars: 3g

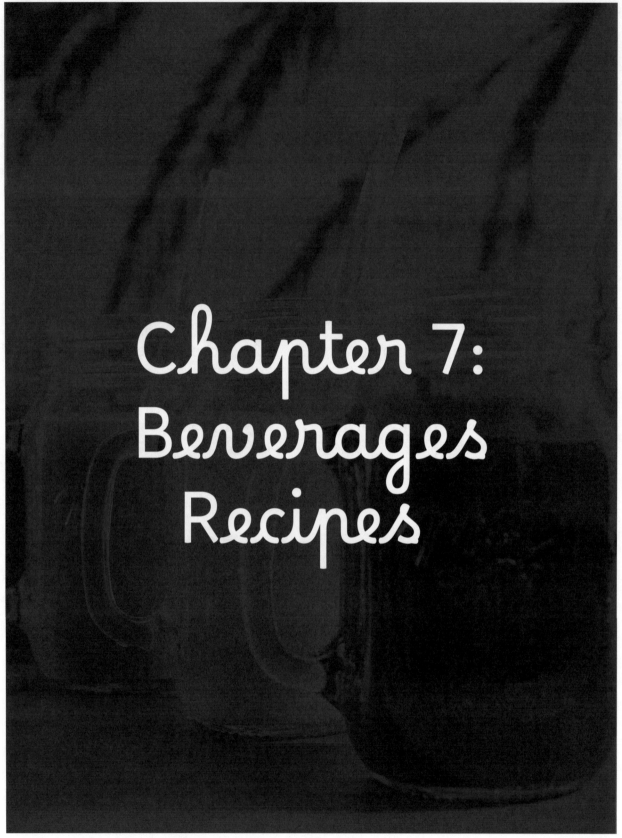

Chapter 7:
Beverages
Recipes

Turmeric Ginger Tea

Prep : 5 min

Serves : 2

Cook: 10 min

Easy

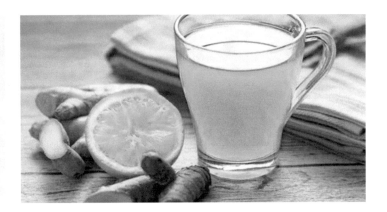

COOKING STEPS

1. In a small saucepan, bring water to a boil.
2. Add turmeric, ginger, and black pepper. Reduce heat and simmer for 10 minutes.
3. Strain the tea into a cup.
4. Stir in honey or maple syrup and lemon juice.
5. Serve hot.

INGREDIENTS

- 2 cups water
- 1 teaspoon ground turmeric
- 1 teaspoon grated fresh ginger
- 1 tablespoon honey or maple syrup
- 1 tablespoon lemon juice
- A pinch of black pepper

- Calories: 40, Protein: 0g, Carbohydrates: 10g, Fiber: 0g, Fat: 0g, Sugars: 9g

Green Smoothie

Prep : 5 min

Serves : 1

Cook : None

Easy

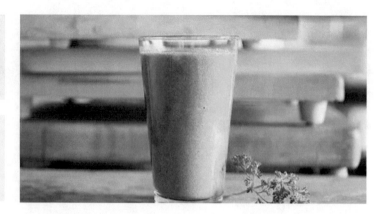

COOKING STEPS

1. Combine all ingredients in a blender.
2. Blend until smooth.
3. Pour into a glass and serve immediately.

INGREDIENTS

- 1 cup spinach
- 1 banana
- 1/2 cup frozen mango chunks
- 1/2 cup almond milk
- 1 tablespoon chia seeds
- 1 tablespoon flax seeds

- Calories: 200, Protein: 5g, Carbohydrates: 38g, Fiber: 8g, Fat: 6g, Sugars: 18g

Golden Milk

Prep : 5 min

Serves : 1

Cook : 5 min

Easy

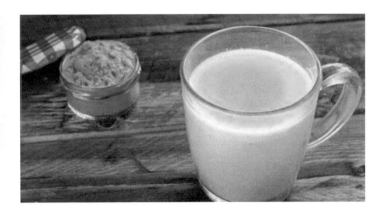

COOKING STEPS

1. In a small saucepan, combine almond milk, turmeric, cinnamon, ginger, and black pepper.
2. Heat over medium heat until warm, stirring occasionally.
3. Remove from heat and stir in honey or maple syrup.
4. Pour into a mug and serve hot.

INGREDIENTS

- 1 cup unsweetened almond milk
- 1 teaspoon ground turmeric
- 1/2 teaspoon ground cinnamon
- 1/4 teaspoon ground ginger
- 1 tablespoon honey or maple syrup
- A pinch of black pepper

- Calories: 100, Protein: 1g, Carbohydrates: 17g, Fiber: 1g, Fat: 3g, Sugars: 13g

Berry Antioxidant Smoothie

  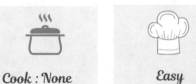 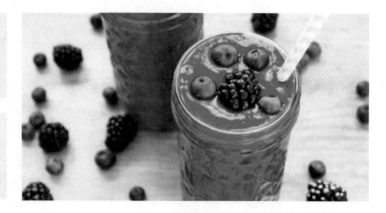

Prep : 5 min

Serves : 1

Cook : None

Easy

COOKING STEPS

1. Combine all ingredients in a blender.
2. Blend until smooth.
3. Pour into a glass and serve immediately.

INGREDIENTS

- 1/2 cup frozen blueberries
- 1/2 cup frozen strawberries
- 1/2 cup Greek yogurt
- 1/2 cup unsweetened almond milk
- 1 tablespoon honey or maple syrup

- Calories: 150, Protein: 8g, Carbohydrates: 27g, Fiber: 4g, Fat: 3g, Sugars: 20g

Matcha Latte

 Prep : 5 min

 Serves : 1

 Cook: 5 min

 Easy

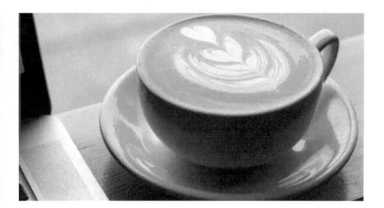

COOKING STEPS

1. In a small saucepan, heat almond milk until warm.
2. Whisk in matcha powder, honey or maple syrup, and vanilla extract until frothy.
3. Pour into a mug and serve hot.

INGREDIENTS

- 1 teaspoon matcha powder
- 1 cup unsweetened almond milk
- 1 tablespoon honey or maple syrup
- 1/2 teaspoon vanilla extract

- Calories: 100, Protein: 1g, Carbohydrates: 18g, Fiber: 1g, Fat: 3g, Sugars: 13g

Cucumber Mint Water

Prep : 5 min

Serves : 8

Cook : None

Easy

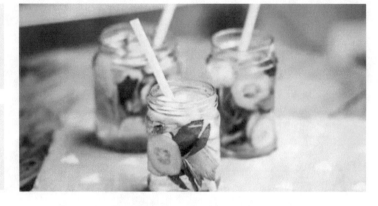

COOKING STEPS

1. In a large pitcher, combine cucumber slices, mint leaves, and lemon slices.
2. Fill with water.
3. Refrigerate for at least 1 hour before serving.

INGREDIENTS

- 1 cucumber, thinly sliced
- 1/4 cup fresh mint leaves
- 1 lemon, sliced
- 8 cups water

- Calories: 5, Protein: 0g Carbohydrates: 1g, Fiber: 0g, Fat: 0g, Sugars: 0g

Beetroot Juice

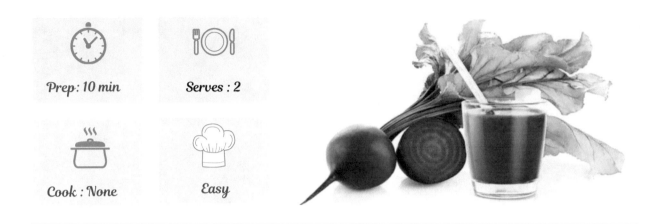

Prep: 10 min

Serves : 2

Cook : None

Easy

COOKING STEPS

1. In a blender, combine beetroots, apple, carrot, lemon juice, and water.
2. Blend until smooth.
3. Strain the mixture through a fine mesh sieve or cheesecloth.
4. Pour into a glass and serve immediately.

INGREDIENTS

- 2 medium beetroots, peeled and chopped
- 1 apple, chopped
- 1 carrot, chopped
- 1 tablespoon lemon juice
- 1 cup water

- Calories: 100, Protein: 2g, Carbohydrates: 25g, Fiber: 5g, Fat: 0g, Sugars: 18g

Pineapple Turmeric Smoothie

Prep : 5 min

Serves : 1

Cook : None

Easy

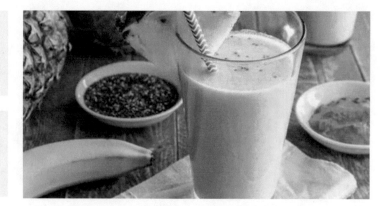

COOKING STEPS

1. Combine all ingredients in a blender.
2. Blend until smooth.
3. Pour into a glass and serve immediately.

INGREDIENTS

- 1 cup frozen pineapple chunks
- 1/2 banana
- 1 cup coconut water
- 1 teaspoon ground turmeric
- 1 teaspoon grated fresh ginger

- Calories: 150, Protein: 1g, Carbohydrates: 36g, Fiber: 4g, Fat: 0g,.Sugars: 27g

Warm Lemon and Ginger Detox Drink

Prep : 5 min

Serves : 2

Cook: 10 min

Easy

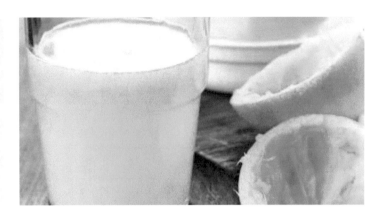

COOKING STEPS

1. In a small saucepan, bring water to a boil.
2. Add lemon juice and ginger slices. Reduce heat and simmer for 10 minutes.
3. Remove from heat and stir in honey or maple syrup.
4. Strain into a cup and serve warm.

INGREDIENTS

- 2 cups water
- 1 lemon, juiced
- 1-inch piece fresh ginger, sliced
- 1 tablespoon honey or maple syrup

- Calories: 30, Protein: 0g, Carbohydrates: 8g, Fiber: 0g, Fat: 0g, Sugars: 7g

Chia Fresca

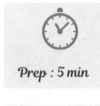

Prep : 5 min

Serves : 2

Cook : None

Easy

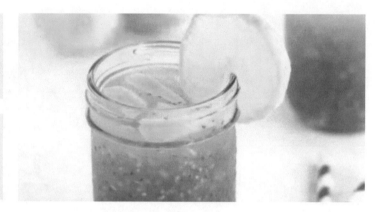

COOKING STEPS

1. In a large glass or jar, combine water, chia seeds, lemon juice, and honey or maple syrup.
2. Stir well and let sit for 10 minutes, stirring occasionally to prevent clumping.
3. Serve chilled.

INGREDIENTS

- 2 cups water
- 1 tablespoon chia seeds
- 1 tablespoon lemon juice
- 1 tablespoon honey or maple syrup

- Calories: 50, Protein: 1g, Carbohydrates: 12g, Fiber: 3g, Fat: 1g, Sugars: 8g

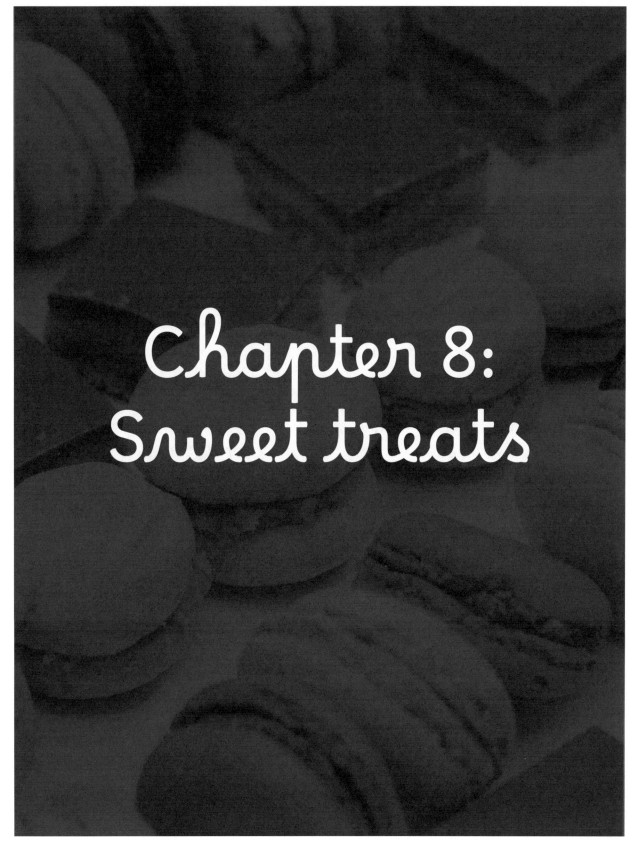

Chapter 8: Sweet treats

Blueberry Chia Pudding

Prep : 5 min

Serves : 2

Cook : None

Easy

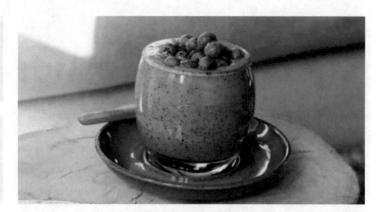

COOKING STEPS

1. In a bowl, whisk together almond milk, chia seeds, honey, and vanilla extract.
2. Cover and refrigerate for at least 4 hours or overnight.
3. Stir the pudding and top with fresh blueberries before serving.

INGREDIENTS

- 1 cup unsweetened almond milk
- 1/4 cup chia seeds
- 1 tablespoon honey or maple syrup
- 1/2 teaspoon vanilla extract
- 1/2 cup fresh blueberries

- Calories: 200, Protein: 6g, Carbohydrates: 28g, Fiber: 11g, Fat: 9g, Sugars: 13g

Dark Chocolate Avocado Mousse

 Prep: 10 min

 Serves : 4

 Cook : None

 Easy

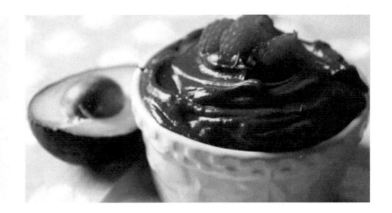

COOKING STEPS

1. In a blender or food processor, combine avocados, cocoa powder, honey, almond milk, vanilla extract, and sea salt.
2. Blend until smooth and creamy.
3. Chill in the refrigerator for at least 30 minutes before serving.

INGREDIENTS

- 2 ripe avocados
- 1/4 cup cocoa powder
- 1/4 cup honey or maple syrup
- 1/4 cup almond milk
- 1 teaspoon vanilla extract
- A pinch of sea salt

- Calories: 250, Protein: 3g, Carbohydrates: 30g, Fiber: 7g, Fat: 15g, Sugars: 20g

Coconut Macaroons

Prep: 10 min

Serves : 12

Cook: 15 min

Easy

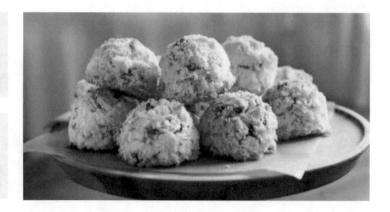

COOKING STEPS

1. Preheat the oven to 350°F (175°C).
2. In a bowl, combine shredded coconut, honey, egg whites, vanilla extract, and sea salt.
3. Drop spoonfuls of the mixture onto a parchment-lined baking sheet.
4. Bake for 15-20 minutes, until golden brown.
5. Cool before serving.

INGREDIENTS

- 2 cups unsweetened shredded coconut
- 1/4 cup honey or maple syrup
- 2 egg whites
- 1 teaspoon vanilla extract
- A pinch of sea salt

- Calories: 100, Protein: 1g, Carbohydrates: 10g, Fiber: 2g, Fat: 6g, Sugars: 8g

Berry Nice Cream

Prep : 5 min

Serves : 2

Cook : None

Easy

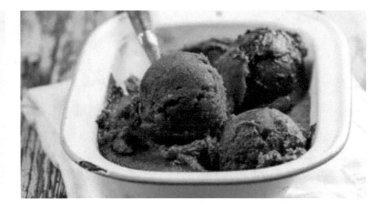

COOKING STEPS

1. In a blender, combine frozen berries, banana, almond milk, and honey.
2. Blend until smooth and creamy.
3. Serve immediately or freeze for a firmer texture.

INGREDIENTS

- 2 cups frozen mixed berries
- 1 frozen banana
- 1/4 cup unsweetened almond milk
- 1 tablespoon honey or maple syrup

- Calories: 150, Protein: 2g, Carbohydrates: 35g, Fiber: 7g, Fat: 1g, Sugars: 22g

Apple Cinnamon Baked Oatmeal Cups

Prep: 10 min

Serves : 12

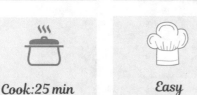
Cook:25 min

Easy

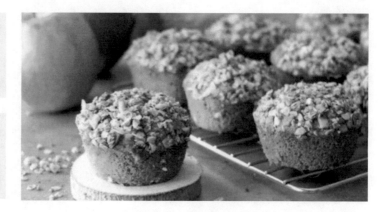

COOKING STEPS

1. Preheat the oven to 350°F (175°C).
2. In a large bowl, mix together oats, cinnamon, baking powder, and salt.
3. Add applesauce, almond milk, honey, vanilla extract, and chopped apple. Stir until well combined.
4. Divide the mixture into a greased muffin tin.
5. Bake for 20-25 minutes, until golden brown and set.
6. Cool before serving.

INGREDIENTS

- 2 cups rolled oats
- 1 teaspoon ground cinnamon
- 1 teaspoon baking powder
- 1/2 teaspoon salt
- 1 cup unsweetened applesauce
- 1/2 cup almond milk
- 1/4 cup honey or maple syrup
- 1 teaspoon vanilla extract
- 1 apple, chopped

- Calories: 100, Protein: 2g, Carbohydrates: 22g, Fiber: 3g, Fat: 1g, Sugars: 10g

Pumpkin Spice Energy Balls

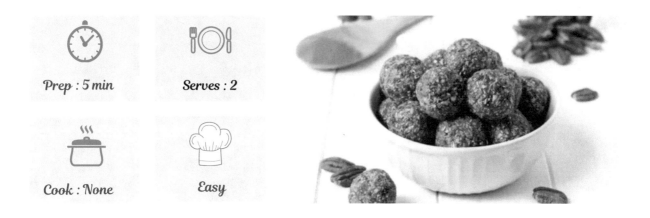

Prep : 5 min

Serves : 2

Cook : None

Easy

COOKING STEPS

1. In a bowl, mix together oats, pumpkin puree, honey, almond butter, and pumpkin pie spice until well combined.
2. Stir in chocolate chips if using.
3. Roll the mixture into 1-inch balls and place on a parchment-lined tray.
4. Refrigerate for at least 30 minutes to firm up.
5. Store in an airtight container in the fridge.

INGREDIENTS

- 1 cup rolled oats
- 1/2 cup canned pumpkin puree
- 1/4 cup honey or maple syrup
- 1/4 cup almond butter
- 1 teaspoon pumpkin pie spice
- 1/4 cup mini dark chocolate chips (optional)

- Calories: 120, Protein: 3g, Carbohydrates: 20g, Fiber: 3g, Fat: 5g, Sugars: 10g

Chia Seed Jam

Prep : 5 min

Serves : 8

Cook: 10 min

Easy

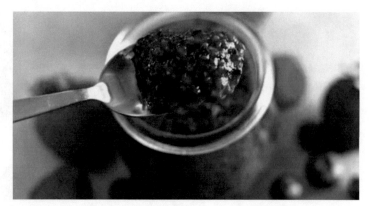

COOKING STEPS

1. In a small saucepan, heat the berries over medium heat until they start to break down, about 5-7 minutes.
2. Mash the berries with a fork or potato masher.
3. Stir in chia seeds, honey, and lemon juice.
4. Cook for an additional 5 minutes, stirring frequently.
5. Remove from heat and let cool. The jam will thicken as it cools.
6. Store in a jar in the refrigerator.

INGREDIENTS

- 2 cups fresh or frozen berries (strawberries, raspberries, blueberries)
- 2 tablespoons chia seeds
- 1-2 tablespoons honey or maple syrup
- 1 teaspoon lemon juice

- Calories: 30, Protein: 1g, Carbohydrates: 6g, Fiber: 3g, Fat: 1g, Sugars: 3g

Banana Oat Cookies

Prep: 10 min

Serves : 12

Cook : 20 mi

Easy

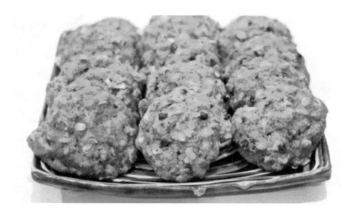

COOKING STEPS

1. Preheat the oven to 350°F (175°C).
2. In a bowl, mix together mashed bananas and rolled oats until well combined.
3. Stir in chocolate chips and nuts if using.
4. Drop spoonfuls of the mixture onto a parchment-lined baking sheet.
5. Bake for 15-20 minutes, until golden brown.
6. Cool before serving.

INGREDIENTS

- 2 ripe bananas, mashed
- 1 cup rolled oats
- 1/4 cup dark chocolate chips (optional)
- 1/4 cup chopped nuts (optional)

- Protein: 1g, Carbohydrates: 14g, Fiber: 2g, Fat: 1g, Sugars: 5g

Mango Coconut Chia Popsicles

Prep: 10 min

Serves : 6

Cook : None

Easy

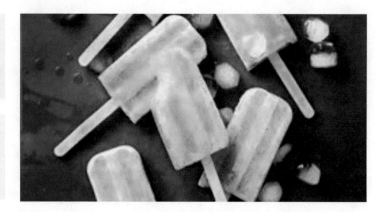

COOKING STEPS

1. In a blender, combine coconut milk, mango chunks, and honey. Blend until smooth.
2. Stir in chia seeds.
3. Pour the mixture into popsicle molds.
4. Freeze for at least 4 hours or until solid.
5. Remove from molds and serve.

INGREDIENTS

- 1 cup coconut milk
- 1 cup fresh or frozen mango chunks
- 1/4 cup chia seeds
- 1-2 tablespoons honey or maple syrup

- Calories: 90, Protein: 1g, Carbohydrates: 14g, Fiber: 3g, Fat: 4g, Sugars: 9g

Cacao Banana Ice Cream

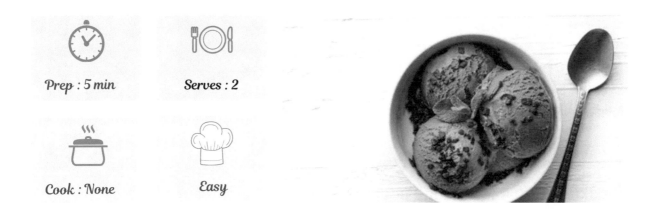

Prep : 5 min

Serves : 2

Cook : None

Easy

COOKING STEPS

1. In a food processor, combine frozen banana slices, cacao powder, almond butter, and honey.
2. Blend until smooth and creamy, scraping down the sides as needed.
3. Serve immediately or freeze for a firmer texture.

INGREDIENTS

- 3 ripe bananas, sliced and frozen
- 2 tablespoons cacao powder
- 1 tablespoon almond butter
- 1 tablespoon honey or maple syrup

- Calories: 180, Protein: 3g, Carbohydrates: 41g, Fiber: 6g, Fat: 4g, Sugars: 27g

Chapter 9: Meal planning and Prep tips

Creating a Weekly Meal Plan

Monday

Breakfast: Blueberry Chia Pudding
Preparation Time: 5 minutes (night before)
Nutritional Information: 200 calories, 6g protein, 28g carbohydrates, 11g fiber, 9g fat, 13g sugars

Lunch: Quinoa Salad with Chickpeas and Avocado
Preparation Time: 10 minutes
Nutritional Information: 350 calories, 12g protein, 45g carbohydrates, 10g fiber, 14g fat, 5g sugars

Dinner: Grilled Salmon with Asparagus
Preparation Time: 10 minutes
Cooking Time: 15 minutes
Nutritional Information: 400 calories, 35g protein, 10g carbohydrates, 5g fiber, 25g fat, 2g sugars

Snack: Pumpkin Spice Energy Balls
Preparation Time: 10 minutes
Nutritional Information: 120 calories, 3g protein, 20g carbohydrates, 3g fiber, 5g fat, 10g sugars

Beverage: Turmeric Ginger Tea
Preparation Time: 5 minutes
Cooking Time: 10 minutes
Nutritional Information: 40 calories, 0g protein, 10g carbohydrates, 0g fiber, 0g fat, 9g sugars

Tuesday

Breakfast: Green Smoothie
Preparation Time: 5 minutes
Nutritional Information: 200 calories, 5g protein, 38g carbohydrates, 8g fiber, 6g fat, 18g sugars

Lunch: Lentil Soup
Preparation Time: 10 minutes
Cooking Time: 20 minutes
Nutritional Information: 300 calories, 18g protein, 45g carbohydrates, 15g fiber, 6g fat, 10g sugars

Dinner: Turkey and Vegetable Stir-Fry
Preparation Time: 10 minutes
Cooking Time: 15 minutes
Nutritional Information: 350 calories, 30g protein, 30g carbohydrates, 5g fiber, 12g fat, 8g sugars

Snack: Banana Oat Cookies
Preparation Time: 10 minutes
Cooking Time: 20 minutes
Nutritional Information: 70 calories, 1g protein, 14g carbohydrates, 2g fiber, 1g fat, 5g sugars

Beverage: Golden Milk
Preparation Time: 5 minutes
Cooking Time: 5 minutes
Nutritional Information: 100 calories, 1g protein, 17g carbohydrates, 1g fiber, 3g fat, 13g sugars

Wednesday

Breakfast: Apple Cinnamon Baked Oatmeal Cups
Preparation Time: 10 minutes
Cooking Time: 25 minutes
Nutritional Information: 100 calories, 2g protein, 22g carbohydrates, 3g fiber, 1g fat, 10g sugars

Lunch: Mediterranean Chickpea Salad
Preparation Time: 10 minutes
Nutritional Information: 350 calories, 12g protein, 40g carbohydrates, 10g fiber, 18g fat, 5g sugars

Dinner: Spaghetti Squash with Marinara Sauce
Preparation Time: 10 minutes
Cooking Time: 40 minutes
Nutritional Information: 300 calories, 10g protein, 45g carbohydrates, 8g fiber, 10g fat, 15g sugars

Snack: Chia Seed Jam with Whole Grain Crackers
Preparation Time: 5 minutes
Cooking Time: 10 minutes
Nutritional Information: 80 calories, 1g protein, 15g carbohydrates, 3g fiber, 2g fat, 8g sugars

Beverage: Berry Antioxidant Smoothie

Preparation Time: 5 minutes

Nutritional Information: 150 calories, 8g protein, 27g carbohydrates, 4g fiber, 3g fat, 20g sugars

Thursday

Breakfast: Cacao Banana Ice Cream

Preparation Time: 5 minutes

Nutritional Information: 180 calories, 3g protein, 41g carbohydrates, 6g fiber, 4g fat, 27g sugars

Lunch: Quinoa and Black Bean Stuffed Peppers

Preparation Time: 10 minutes

Cooking Time: 30 minutes

Nutritional Information: 300 calories, 10g protein, 45g carbohydrates, 12g fiber, 8g fat, 10g sugars

Dinner: Lemon Garlic Shrimp with Zucchini Noodles

Preparation Time: 10 minutes

Cooking Time: 10 minutes

Nutritional Information: 350 calories, 30g protein, 20g carbohydrates, 4g fiber, 15g fat, 8g sugars

Snack: Mango Coconut Chia Popsicles

Preparation Time: 10 minutes

Nutritional Information: 90 calories, 1g protein, 14g carbohydrates, 3g fiber, 4g fat, 9g sugars

Beverage: Matcha Latte
Preparation Time: 5 minutes
Cooking Time: 5 minutes
Nutritional Information: 100 calories, 1g protein, 18g carbohydrates, 1g fiber, 3g fat, 13g sugars

Friday

Breakfast: Dark Chocolate Avocado Mousse
Preparation Time: 10 minutes
Nutritional Information: 250 calories, 3g protein, 30g carbohydrates, 7g fiber, 15g fat, 20g sugars

Lunch: Grilled Chicken Salad with Avocado and Mango
Preparation Time: 10 minutes
Cooking Time: 10 minutes
Nutritional Information: 400 calories, 30g protein, 30g carbohydrates, 8g fiber, 18g fat, 15g sugars

Dinner: Baked Cod with Sweet Potato Fries
Preparation Time: 10 minutes
Cooking Time: 25 minutes
Nutritional Information: 350 calories, 30g protein, 40g carbohydrates, 6g fiber, 10g fat, 10g sugars

Snack: Coconut Macaroons
Preparation Time: 10 minutes
Cooking Time: 15 minutes
Nutritional Information: 100 calories, 1g protein, 10g carbohydrates, 2g fiber, 6g fat, 8g sugars

Beverage: Pineapple Turmeric Smoothie

Preparation Time: 5 minutes

Nutritional Information: 150 calories, 1g protein, 36g carbohydrates, 4g fiber, 0g fat, 27g sugars

Saturday

Breakfast: Berry Nice Cream

Preparation Time: 5 minutes

Nutritional Information: 150 calories, 2g protein, 35g carbohydrates, 7g fiber, 1g fat, 22g sugars

Lunch: Spinach and Quinoa Stuffed Portobello Mushrooms

Preparation Time: 10 minutes

Cooking Time: 25 minutes

Nutritional Information: 300 calories, 12g protein, 45g carbohydrates, 10g fiber, 10g fat, 8g sugars

Dinner: Chicken and Vegetable Kebabs

Preparation Time: 10 minutes

Cooking Time: 15 minutes

Nutritional Information: 350 calories, 30g protein, 25g carbohydrates, 5g fiber, 15g fat, 10g sugars

Snack: Chia Fresca

Preparation Time: 5 minutes

Nutritional Information: 50 calories, 1g protein, 12g carbohydrates, 3g fiber, 1g fat, 8g sugars

Beverage: Cucumber Mint Water
Preparation Time: 5 minutes
Nutritional Information: 5 calories, 0g protein, 1g carbohydrates, 0g fiber, 0g fat, 0g sugars

Saturday

Breakfast: Berry Nice Cream
Preparation Time: 5 minutes
Nutritional Information: 150 calories, 2g protein, 35g carbohydrates, 7g fiber, 1g fat, 22g sugars

Lunch: Spinach and Quinoa Stuffed Portobello Mushrooms
Preparation Time: 10 minutes
Cooking Time: 25 minutes
Nutritional Information: 300 calories, 12g protein, 45g carbohydrates, 10g fiber, 10g fat, 8g sugars

Dinner: Chicken and Vegetable Kebabs
Preparation Time: 10 minutes
Cooking Time: 15 minutes
Nutritional Information: 350 calories, 30g protein, 25g carbohydrates, 5g fiber, 15g fat, 10g sugars

Snack: Chia Fresca
Preparation Time: 5 minutes
Nutritional Information: 50 calories, 1g protein, 12g carbohydrates, 3g fiber, 1g fat, 8g sugars

Beverage: Cucumber Mint Water
Preparation Time: 5 minutes
Nutritional Information: 5 calories, 0g protein, 1g carbohydrates, 0g fiber, 0g fat, 0g sugars

Sunday

Breakfast: Overnight Oats with Berries and Almonds
Preparation Time: 5 minutes (night before)
Nutritional Information: 250 calories, 8g protein, 40g carbohydrates, 8g fiber, 8g fat, 12g sugars

Lunch: Roasted Veggie and Hummus Wrap
Preparation Time: 10 minutes
Nutritional Information: 300 calories, 10g protein, 45g carbohydrates, 10g fiber, 10g fat, 8g sugars

Dinner: Beef and Broccoli Stir-Fry
Preparation Time: 10 minutes
Cooking Time: 15 minutes
Nutritional Information: 400 calories, 30g protein, 35g carbohydrates, 6g fiber, 15g fat, 10g sugars

Snack: Beetroot Juice
Preparation Time: 10 minutes
Nutritional Information: 100 calories, 2g protein, 25g carbohydrates, 5g fiber, 0g fat, 18g sugars

Beverage: Warm Lemon and Ginger Detox Drink

Preparation Time: 5 minutes

Cooking Time: 10 minutes

Nutritional Information: 30 calories, 0g protein, 8g carbohydrates, 0g fiber, 0g fat, 7g sugars

Batch Cooking for Busy Days

Batch cooking is an excellent strategy for busy days. It allows you to prepare multiple meals in advance, ensuring you have healthy, anti-inflammatory options ready to go. Here's a guide to batch cooking, along with some recipes to get you started.

Benefits of Batch Cooking

Time-Saving: Cook once, eat multiple times.

Convenience: Have ready-made meals on hand.

Cost-Effective: Buy ingredients in bulk.

Healthier Choices: Control ingredients and portion sizes.

Tips for Successful Batch Cooking

Plan Your Meals: Decide on a few recipes you want to prepare.

Make a Grocery List: Include all necessary ingredients.

Choose the Right Containers: Use airtight, BPA-free containers for storage.

Label and Date: Clearly mark what each container holds and when it was made.

Utilize Freezer Space: Freeze portions that you won't consume within a few days.

Batch Cooking Recipes

1. Lentil and Vegetable Soup

Ingredients:
1 cup dried lentils, rinsed
1 onion, diced
2 carrots, chopped
2 celery stalks, chopped
4 cloves garlic, minced
1 can diced tomatoes
6 cups vegetable broth
1 tsp cumin
1 tsp paprika
Salt and pepper to taste
2 cups spinach, chopped

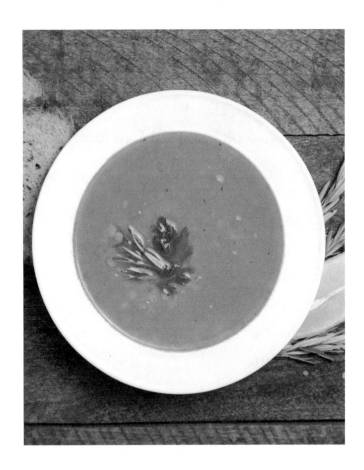

Instructions:
In a large pot, sauté onion, carrots, celery, and garlic until softened.
Stir in lentils, diced tomatoes, paprika, cumin, and salt & pepper.
After reaching a boil, lower the heat, and simmer for 30 to 35 minutes.
Stir in spinach and cook for an additional 5 minutes.

Nutritional Information (per serving, makes 6 servings):
Calories: 180, Protein: 9g, Carbohydrates: 30g, Fiber: 10g, Fat: 2g, Sugars: 8g

Preparation Time: 15 minutes
Cooking Time: 40 minutes
Serving: 6

2. Chicken and Vegetable Stir-Fry

Ingredients:

2 lbs boneless, skinless chicken breasts, sliced

2 bell peppers, sliced

1 large broccoli head, cut into florets

2 carrots, sliced, 1 onion, sliced

4 cloves garlic, minced

1/4 cup soy sauce (low sodium)

2 tbsp olive oil

1 tsp ginger, grated

2 tbsp honey or maple syrup

1 tbsp cornstarch (optional for thickening)

1/4 cup water

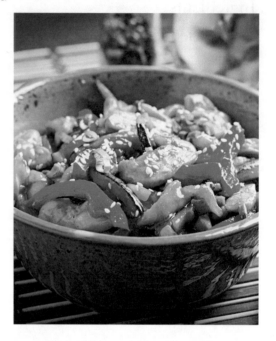

Instructions:

In a large pan, heat olive oil and cook chicken until browned. Remove and set aside.

Add the veggies, ginger, and garlic to the same pan. Cook until tender-crisp. Return chicken to the pan.

In a small bowl, mix soy sauce, honey, water, and cornstarch. Pour over chicken and vegetables.

Cook for an additional 5 minutes until sauce thickens.

Nutritional Information (per serving, makes 6 servings):

Calories: 300, Protein: 30g, Carbohydrates: 15g, Fiber: 4g, Fat: 12g, Sugars: 8g

Preparation Time: 15 minutes

Cooking Time: 20 minutes

Serving: 6

3. Quinoa and Black Bean Salad

Ingredients:
1 cup quinoa, rinsed
1 can black beans, drained and rinsed
1 red bell pepper, diced
1 cup corn kernels (fresh or frozen)
1/4 cup red onion, finely chopped
1/4 cup fresh cilantro, chopped
1/4 cup olive oil
2 tbsp lime juice
1 tsp cumin
Salt and pepper to taste

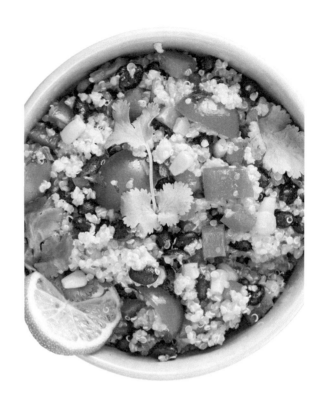

Instructions:
Cook quinoa according to package instructions. Let cool.
In a large bowl, combine quinoa, black beans, bell pepper, corn, onion, and cilantro.
Mix the olive oil, lime juice, cumin, salt, and pepper in a small bowl. Drizzle over the salad and mix thoroughly.

Nutritional Information (per serving, makes 4 servings):
Calories: 250, Protein: 8g, Carbohydrates: 40g, Fiber: 8g, Fat: 10g, Sugars: 4g

Preparation Time: 15 minutes
Cooking Time: 15 minutes
Serving: 4

4. Baked Turkey Meatballs

Ingredients:

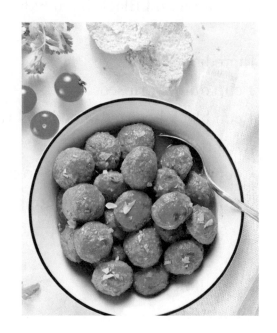

1 lb ground turkey

1/2 cup breadcrumbs (whole grain)

1/4 cup grated Parmesan cheese

1 egg

2 cloves garlic, minced

1 tsp Italian seasoning

Salt and pepper to taste

Instructions:

Preheat the oven to 375°F (190°C).

Mix all the ingredients together in a big bowl.

Shape into meatballs measuring one inch, then transfer to a baking sheet covered with parchment paper.

Bake for 20-25 minutes, until cooked through.

Nutritional Information (per serving, makes 4 servings):

Calories: 220, Protein: 28g, Carbohydrates: 8g, Fiber: 1g, Fat: 8g, Sugars: 1g

Preparation Time: 10 minutes

Cooking Time: 25 minutes

Serving: 4

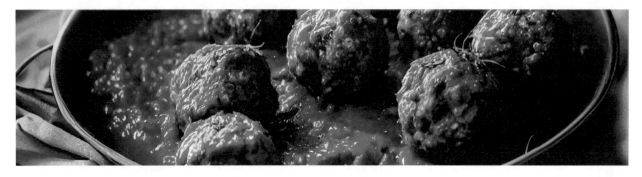

5. Sweet Potato and Chickpea Curry

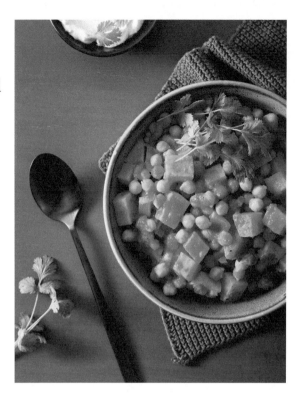

Ingredients:
2 large sweet potatoes, peeled and cubed
1 can chickpeas, drained and rinsed
1 onion, diced
3 cloves garlic, minced
1 can coconut milk
1 can diced tomatoes
2 tbsp curry powder
1 tsp cumin
1 tsp turmeric
Salt and pepper to taste
2 cups spinach, chopped

Instructions:
Add the onion and garlic to a large pot and sauté until softened.
Add sweet potatoes, chickpeas, coconut milk, diced tomatoes, curry powder, cumin, turmeric, salt, and pepper.
Bring to a boil, then reduce heat and simmer for 20-25 minutes, until sweet potatoes are tender.
Stir in spinach and cook for an additional 5 minutes.

Nutritional Information (per serving, makes 6 servings):
Calories: 300, Protein: 8g, Carbohydrates: 50g, Fiber: 10g, Fat: 10g, Sugars: 12g
Preparation Time: 15 minutes
Cooking Time: 30 minutes
Serving: 6

6. Overnight Oats with Berries and Almonds

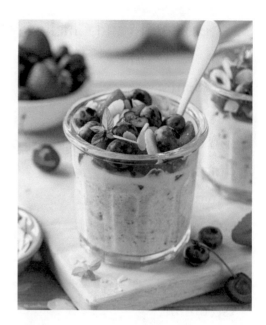

Ingredients:

2 cups rolled oats

2 cups unsweetened almond milk

1 cup fresh or frozen berries

1/4 cup almonds, chopped

2 tbsp chia seeds

2 tbsp honey or maple syrup

Instructions:

In a large bowl, combine oats, almond milk, berries, almonds, chia seeds, and honey.

Mix well and divide into individual jars or containers.

Refrigerate overnight and enjoy in the morning.

Nutritional Information (per serving, makes 4 servings):

Calories: 250,.Protein: 6g, Carbohydrates: 40g, Fiber: 8g,.Fat: 8g, Sugars: 12g

Preparation Time: 10 minutes

Cooking Time: None (refrigerate overnight)

Serving: 4

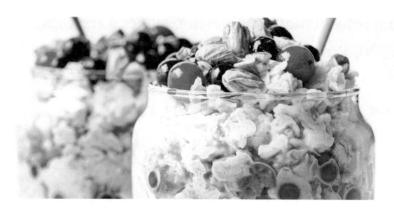

7. Vegetable Frittata

Ingredients:
8 eggs
1/4 cup milk (dairy or non-dairy)
1 cup spinach, chopped
1 bell pepper, diced
1/2 onion, diced
1/2 cup cherry tomatoes, halved
1/4 cup feta cheese, crumbled
Salt and pepper to taste
1 tbsp olive oil

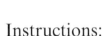

Instructions:
Preheat the oven to 350°F (175°C).

Whisk the eggs and milk together in a big bowl. Season with salt and pepper.

In an oven-safe skillet, heat olive oil and sauté spinach, bell pepper, and onion until softened.

Pour egg mixture over vegetables and sprinkle with cherry tomatoes and feta cheese.

Cook on the stovetop for 5 minutes, then transfer to the oven and bake for 20-25 minutes, until set.

Nutritional Information (per serving, makes 4 servings):
Calories: 200, Protein: 12g, Carbohydrates: 8g, Fiber: 2g, Fat: 14g, Sugars: 4g

Preparation Time: 10 minutes
Cooking Time: 25 minutes
Serving: 4

8. Homemade Granola

Ingredients:
3 cups rolled oats
One cup of chopped nuts (almonds, walnuts, or pecans)
1/2 cup dried fruit (raisins, cranberries, or apricots), chopped
1/4 cup honey or maple syrup
1/4 cup coconut oil, melted
1 tsp vanilla extract
1 tsp cinnamon
1/4 tsp salt

Instructions:
Preheat the oven to 300°F (150°C).
In a large bowl, combine oats, nuts, dried fruit, honey, coconut oil, vanilla extract, cinnamon, and salt. Mix well.
Evenly distribute the ingredients onto a parchment paper-lined baking sheet.
Bake until golden brown, stirring every 25 to 30 minutes.
Before storing in an airtight container, allow it to cool fully

Nutritional Information (per serving, makes 10 servings):
Calories: 200, Protein: 4g, Carbohydrates: 28g, Fiber: 4g, Fat: 10g, Sugars: 12g

Preparation Time: 10 minutes
Cooking Time: 30 minutes
Serving: 10

9. Roasted Vegetables

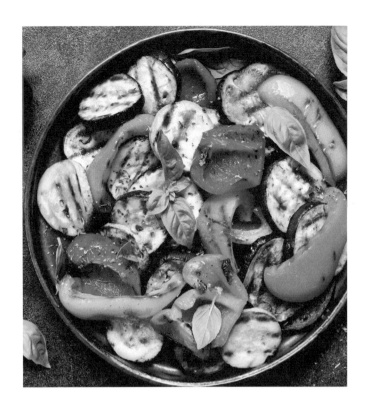

Ingredients:
2 carrots, chopped
1 sweet potato, cubed
1 red bell pepper, chopped
1 zucchini, sliced
1 red onion, chopped
2 tbsp olive oil
1 tsp garlic powder
1 tsp paprika
Salt and pepper to taste

Instructions:
Preheat the oven to 400°F (200°C).
Combine the vegetables, paprika, garlic powder, salt, and pepper in a big bowl.
Arrange the vegetables on a parchment paper-lined baking sheet.
Roast for 25 to 30 minutes, or until soft and browned.

Nutritional Information (per serving, makes 4 servings):
Calories: 150,.Protein: 2g, Carbohydrates: 20g, Fiber: 5g, Fat: 7g, Sugars: 8g

Preparation Time: 10 minutes
Cooking Time: 30 minutes
Serving: 4

10. Stuffed Bell Peppers

Ingredients:
4 bell peppers with the tops removed and the seeds extracted
1 cup cooked quinoa
1 can black beans, drained and rinsed
1 cup corn kernels (fresh or frozen)
1/2 onion, diced
1 tsp cumin
1 tsp chili powder
Salt and pepper to taste
1/2 cup shredded cheese (optional)

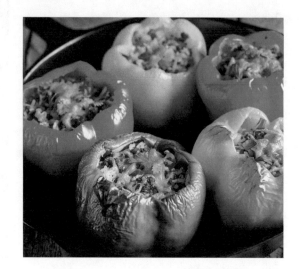

Instructions:
Preheat the oven to 375°F (190°C).
In a large bowl, combine quinoa, black beans, corn, onion, cumin, chili powder, salt, and pepper.
Stuff bell peppers with quinoa mixture and place in a baking dish.
If using, sprinkle cheese on top of each stuffed pepper.
Cover with foil and bake for 30 minutes.Take off the foil and continue baking for ten more minutes.

Nutritional Information (per serving, makes 4 servings):
Calories: 250, Protein: 10g, Carbohydrates: 45g, Fiber: 12g, Fat: 5g, Sugars: 8g

Preparation Time: 15 minutes
Cooking Time: 40 minutes
Serving: 4

Storing and Reheating Tips

Proper storage and reheating are crucial for maintaining the quality and safety of your batch-cooked meals. Here are some guidelines to help you store and reheat your meals effectively:

Storing Tips

Use Appropriate Containers:
Opt for airtight containers made of glass or BPA-free plastic to keep food fresh and prevent contamination.
Choose containers of various sizes for different portions, making it easy to grab a single serving.

Label and Date:
Clearly label each container with the contents and the date it was prepared. This helps you keep track of what needs to be eaten first and ensures you don't consume food past its safe storage period.

Cool Before Storing:
Allow hot food to cool to room temperature before refrigerating or freezing. This prevents condensation, which can cause food to become soggy and spoil faster.

Refrigeration:
Store perishable foods in the refrigerator for up to 3-4 days. Items like cooked meats, grains, and vegetables should be consumed within this time frame to ensure safety and quality.

Freezing:

For longer storage, freeze meals in portion-sized containers. Most cooked foods can be safely frozen for 2-3 months.

To avoid freezer burn, use heavy-duty freezer bags or freezer-safe containers.

Leave some space at the top of containers to allow for expansion as the food freezes.

Reheating Tips

Thaw Safely:

Thaw frozen meals in the refrigerator overnight for best results.

For quicker thawing, use the microwave's defrost function or place the container in a bowl of cold water. Never thaw food at room temperature as it increases the risk of bacterial growth.

Microwave Reheating:

Transfer food to a microwave-safe container if it's not already in one.

Cover with a microwave-safe lid or wrap to retain moisture and ensure even heating.

Stir food halfway through heating to promote even temperature distribution.

Use the microwave's reheat function or heat in short intervals, checking and stirring between intervals.

Stovetop Reheating:

For soups, stews, and curries, reheat in a saucepan over medium heat, stirring occasionally until heated through.

Add a splash of water or broth if the food has thickened too much during storage.

Oven Reheating:

Preheat the oven to 350°F (175°C).

Transfer food to an oven-safe dish and cover with foil to prevent drying out.

Reheat for 20-30 minutes, depending on the type and quantity of food. Check to ensure it's heated evenly.

Reheating Vegetables:

Avoid overcooking vegetables during reheating as they can become mushy.

Reheat quickly in a skillet with a small amount of olive oil or in the microwave for 1-2 minutes.

Tips for Maintaining Quality

Avoid Multiple Reheatings:

Reheat only the portion you plan to eat to preserve the quality of the remaining food.

Repeated reheating can degrade the taste and texture of food and increase the risk of bacterial growth.

Check for Freshness:

Always smell and visually inspect food before reheating. Discard any food that shows signs of spoilage, such as off smells, discoloration, or mold.

Add Fresh Ingredients:

Enhance reheated meals by adding fresh herbs, a squeeze of lemon, or a drizzle of olive oil to brighten flavors.

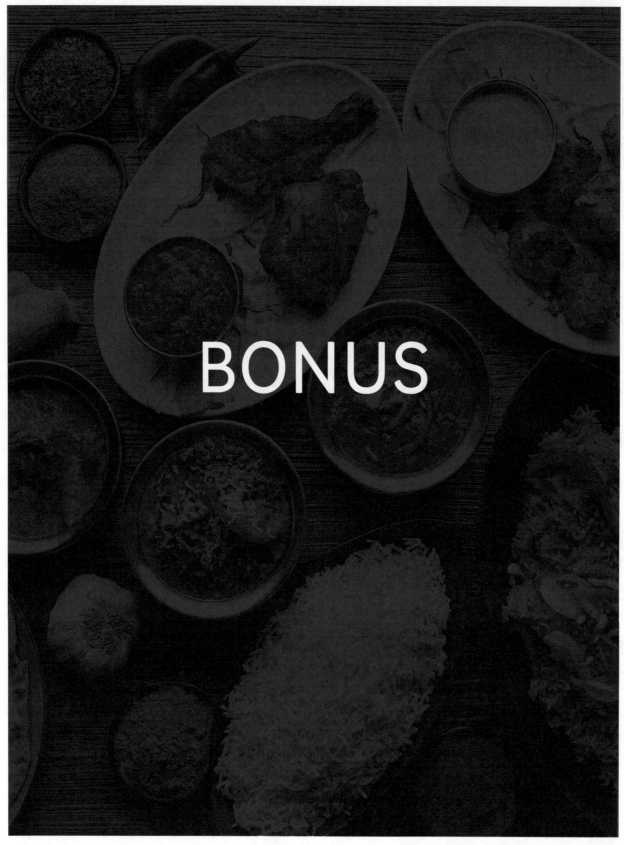

BONUS

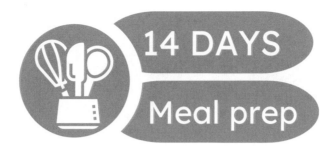

14 DAYS Meal prep

WEEK 1

	Breakfast	Lunch	Dinner
M	Yogurt, Honey, Chia	Quinoa Veggie Salad	Baked Salmon, Sweet Potatoes, Broccoli
T	Oatmeal with Berries	Egg Salad	Carrots, Hummus
W	Smoothie Bowl	Chicken Caesar Salad	Stir-Fry Veggies, Rice
T	Avocado Toast	Berry Parfait	Grilled Chicken, Quinoa
F	Tuna Salad	Hummus Veggie Wrap	Almonds
S	Chia Pudding	Turkey Avocado Wrap	Turkey Meatballs, Zoodles
S	Spinach, Strawberry Salad	Baked Cod, Asparagus	Shrimp Tacos

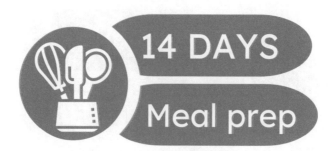

WEEK 2

	Breakfast	**Lunch**	**Dinner**
M	Scrambled Eggs	Caprese Salad	Mixed Berries
T	Veggie Sushi	Quinoa Tabbouleh	Apple Slices
W	Chicken Salad	Grilled Salmon, Kale	Cucumber Slices
T	Banana Smoothie	Beef Stir-Fry, Brown Rice	Stuffed Peppers
F	Omelette, Spinach	Chicken, Veggie Skewers	Shrimp Salad
S	French Toast	Black Bean Chili	Greek Salad
S	Yogurt, Granola	Turkey, Spinach Salad	Pear, Cheese

Conclusion

Embarking on an anti-inflammatory diet journey can seem daunting at first, but with the right recipes and a bit of planning, it becomes not only manageable but also enjoyable. The super easy anti-inflammatory recipes we've explored in this collection are designed to seamlessly integrate into your daily routine, offering a blend of simplicity, nutrition, and flavor. By focusing on fresh, whole ingredients and minimizing processed foods, these recipes support your body's natural ability to reduce inflammation, promoting overall health and well-being.

Adopting an anti-inflammatory diet doesn't mean sacrificing taste or spending hours in the kitchen. From hearty breakfasts to satisfying dinners, and even indulgent desserts, these recipes provide a variety of options that cater to diverse palates and dietary needs. The emphasis on fruits, vegetables, lean proteins, healthy fats, and whole grains ensures that each meal is balanced and nutrient-dense.

Beyond the immediate benefits of reduced inflammation, this dietary approach can contribute to long-term health improvements. Many individuals report enhanced energy levels, improved digestion, and better weight management. Additionally, the anti-inflammatory diet has been linked to a lower risk of chronic diseases such as heart disease, diabetes, and certain cancers.

As you incorporate these super easy anti-inflammatory recipes into your routine, remember that consistency is key. Small, sustainable changes often lead to the most significant results. Feel free to experiment with the recipes, adjusting them to your taste and dietary preferences. The goal is to find a rhythm that works for you and makes healthy eating a pleasurable and integral part of your lifestyle.

Made in United States
Troutdale, OR
10/10/2024